"SIX PRACTICAL LESSONS FOR AN EASIER CHILDBIRTH

is the only book on the Lamaze method of psycho-prophylactic childbirth which clearly and forcefully describes and teaches this method in detail. No one is better qualified to present these lessons than Elisabeth Bing, *the* outstanding teacher and pioneer of the method in the country. No one who reads her book—made vivid through brilliant photographs and exposition—can fail to grasp the method for himself."

—Ralph M. Crowley, M.D.
President, The American Academy of Psychoanalysis

"I am not suprised that this is an exceptional book, for its author is an exceptional woman. Her sincere and personal interest in making childbirth a fulfilling and radiant experience for every woman illuminates each page. I feel certain that these SIX LESSONS will become the bible for many young couples."

—Alan F. Guttmacher, M.D.
former President, Planned Parenthood Federation

Bantam Books by Elisabeth Bing

MOVING THROUGH PREGNANCY
SIX PRACTICAL LESSONS FOR AN EASIER
CHILDBIRTH

SIX PRACTICAL LESSONS FOR AN EASIER CHILDBIRTH

Revised Edition

by Elisabeth Bing, R.P.T.

Photographs by Norman McGrath
Drawings by Howard S. Friedman

BANTAM BOOKS · TORONTO · NEW YORK · LONDON

SIX PRACTICAL LESSONS FOR AN EASIER CHILDBIRTH

A Bantam Book | published by arrangement with the author

PRINTING HISTORY

Grosset edition published March 1967

2nd printing .... March 1969   3rd printing .... June 1969

An excerpt appeared in EXPECTING under the title "The Lamaze Method" 1967

Bantam edition | October 1969

2nd printing .... April 1970   6th printing .... March 1972
3rd printing .... November 1970   7th printing .... October 1972
4th printing .... June 1971   8th printing .... April 1973
5th printing .... November 1971   9th printing .... November 1973

Revised Bantam edition | March 1977

The author and publisher thank Bill and Gail Meckel for their good-natured assistance in the preparation of this book.

ISBN 0–553–10420–9

Published simultaneously in the United States and Canada

PRINTED IN THE UNITED STATES OF AMERICA

0 9 8 7 6 5 4 3 2 1

This book is dedicated to all the young parents
who have studied with me, and to the
memory of Marjorie Karmel.

Introduction

I wrote the first edition of this book exactly ten years ago, and not in my wildest dreams would I have ever thought that years later, this little textbook could still be in demand and be of practical help to thousands of young parents. Of course, I personally was convinced of the value of the Lamaze method but had simply hoped that "Prepared Childbirth" was here to stay and that its obvious appeal to parents would establish it as a "way of birth," not as some kind of fad of the sixties.

The Lamaze method has now become an accepted modality of obstetric procedure in our time. Today, hardly anyone will argue that it is detrimental to a woman's health or could endanger the newborn. And just because it has proved to be of lasting value, it has also proved to be a living tool. Changes have occurred, changes in technique to some extent, changes in approach, changes in obstetric knowledge; it is as if the infant Lamaze method has grown into early adulthood and that its existence is now taken for granted.

I had been asked for a number of years by many of my colleagues and also by my students, to revise this basic textbook, to bring it up to date (with completely new photographs of the exercises) and to reflect present obstetrical thinking. I would like to thank my editor at Bantam Books, Grace Bechtold, for helping me to describe these changes and to convince Bantam to publish this "growing child" so that it can be of as much help today to as many or more young parents as it has been for the last ten years.

Contents

what to do with your hands; hyperventilation;
the position of your body during early labor;
the husband's role during practice at home.

LESSON 4

Review; back labor; ways to alleviate back
labor; the second breathing technique; using the
second breathing technique in labor; how your
husband can simulate a contraction; the transition;
the technique of breathing during transition.

LESSON 5

Review; the second stage of labor, or "expulsion";
the preliminary expulsion exercises;
what happens during actual delivery;
an exercise to prepare for delivery; the husband's
role during expulsion; the delivery-room table;
how to stop pushing on command.

LESSON 6

Recognizing the first signs of real labor;
breaking of waters; what to do when contractions
begin; what to take to the hospital; arriving
at the hospital; breathing with your labor;
the use of medication; beginning to push;
your baby arrives; after you've given birth.

A Mother's Report

A Father's Report

Foreword

Having begun obstetrics more than forty years ago, I have been privileged to witness a revolution in both its practice and its art. The revolution in practice was brought about through the wider use of prenatal care, transfusion and diagnostic X-ray, and by the introduction of improved anesthesia, better surgical techniques, chemotherapeutics and antibiotics. These improvements in practice produced a startling reduction in illness and death. In my early years we witnessed sixty-seven mothers die per ten thousand births; today less than three deaths occur in ten thousand births.

Change in the art has transformed childbirth from a grim, frightening experience into a happy, cheerful event. One may question why the change did not come sooner. Perhaps because the danger intrinsic in childbirth caused a fanatical concentration on safe deliverance. Then, when safety was accomplished, medicine relaxed its single focus and began to view the non-organic, the psychological aspects of childbirth. Grantly Dick-Read deserves credit for first emphasizing the harmful effects of fear and ignorance, both of which he attempted to dispel. His introduction of natural childbirth was a pioneering step and his sympathetic, tender and somewhat fatherly attitude toward the pregnant woman even overflowed into doctrinaire obstetrics.

The contributions of Lamaze and his disciples have further enriched the welfare of the parturient. By way of parenthesis, I should like to say that I met Dr. Lamaze at his Metal Workers' Hospital in Paris. He was a very large man, almost elephantine in appearance, yet seemed gentle and kind. Despite the language barrier, he took much time and great pains to tell me about his *work.* It is not my purpose to explain the theory or practice of psychoprophylaxis, for Mrs. Bing in her *Six Practical Lessons For An Easier Childbirth* has done this incredibly well, far better than could I or anyone else. I am not surprised that this is an exceptional book, for its author is an exceptional woman. Her sincere and personal interest in making childbirth a fulfilling and radiant experience for every woman illuminates each page.

I feel certain that these *Six Lessons* will become a bible for many young couples. How lucky they are to find it together, for if both study and follow its directions, their joint entrance into parenthood will almost certainly be a triumphant success. Having been a co-worker of the author, I am especially pleased that her personality—rare spirituality and great humanity—comes through to the reader.

Alan F. Guttmacher, M.D.
died March 18, 1974
President, Planned Parenthood Federation
Formerly Chief of Obstetrics and Gynecology,
Mt. Sinai Hospital, New York City

Preface

This book begins where most books on childbirth and maternity end. Other teachers are content to romanticize the glorious aspects of childbearing, to acquaint you with the physiology of pregnancy, to explain fetal growth with beautiful pictures and to describe the mechanism of labor. Mrs. Bing's book, however, has a single aim: to teach you a method by which you can give birth by your own efforts.

Childbirth is one of the most stressful situations in human life. Childbirth demands an immense effort, comparable to the energy expended in a twelve-mile hike. Education that is limited to the physiology of pregnancy and the stages of labor can be compared to knowledge by map alone of a road on which you have to walk. Even if you know the map by heart, that information will not give you the physical training and stamina necessary to perform the hike. In labor, also, intellectual understanding is not enough. When you feel the oncoming uterine contraction—a totally new sensation—your first reaction may be to run away, to panic. Only the discipline imposed by an adequate training can prepare you to cope confidently and without apprehension with this task. You must learn to analyze the changing nature of the uterine contractions, adapt your body to these changes, and respond to them with appropriate breathing techniques.

Mrs. Bing can help you to do just this. But—a fair warning–it is not enough to understand the nature of these exercises; you must practice and practice until you can perform them automatically when you are in labor. Get your husband to coach you every evening until you are both letter-perfect in the method. Many hospitals today permit the husband to stay with his wife during the hours of labor and delivery.

Our technique is called the Lamaze Method, named after the famous obstetrician, Dr. Fernand Lamaze, who first introduced it in France in 1951. The technical name is the Psychoprophylactic Method of Childbirth, which means prevention or lessening of pain by psychological and physical means. The Lamaze Method does not believe in solitary mothers. You should be assisted and encouraged by the team surrounding you: the doctor, your husband, and the nurse.

By thoroughly mastering the method set forth in this book, you can participate actively in the birth of your baby—an experience you will never forget.

Heinz L. Luschinsky, M.D., F.A.C.O.G.

SIX PRACTICAL LESSONS FOR AN EASIER CHILDBIRTH

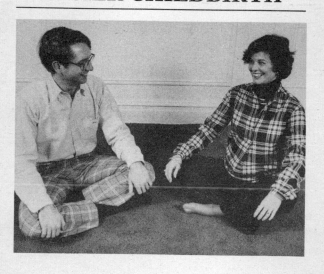

OUR CLASS CONVENES

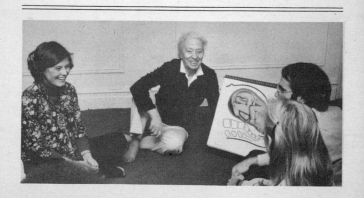

Women all over the world are preparing themselves for childbirth in a new and constructive way. They're learning about the changes that occur in the body during the nine months of gestation; they are doing exercises to prepare their bodies for giving birth; they are practicing new techniques of breathing and relaxation, which will help them ease pain and discomfort during labor and delivery.

This new method of preparation is an intelligent woman's approach to the difficult emotional and physical task of giving birth. Many such women—and their partners—are now taking classes similar to those presented here, but this book will allow prospective parents to prepare for childbirth at home, without any formal curriculum. Our book may be used as a supplement and guide to classes, but its primary value should be as a complete and thorough home course.

To make things as simple and useful as possible, let us begin together as if you were all attending the classes I have given thousands of parents-to-be. If you follow the course closely, practicing the exercises and using the techniques prescribed, I am sure you will have an active, happy and rewarding experience together.

AN INTRODUCTION TO THE LESSONS

You are one of a group of five young couples arriving at my studio for your first lesson. The young women have various occupations: One is a dancer, on leave from a Broadway show; another is a secretary in a law office; the third is a schoolteacher; and there are two housewives, one of whom already has a little boy. The men's professions are varied: a lawyer, a book salesman, a broker, a mechanic, and a graduate student. All that these people have in common is their youth and the fact that each of them will be the parent of a new baby within the next two months.

We have found that the best time to start our course is toward the end of the seventh or the beginning of the eighth month, when a woman is psychologically ready to train herself for labor and delivery. She is beginning to feel the weight of her baby; she may have backaches; her abdominal muscles may feel weak. At this point she is more likely to accept and welcome the idea of training herself for the task ahead. If she had started too early in her pregnancy, the will to work hard at her exercises would very likely have diminished as the months wore on. Intensive training during the last phases of pregnancy not only provides the best physical preparation, but keeps methods and techniques fresh in the mind as actual labor and delivery arrive.

None of us in our class has met the others before, so there is a certain feeling of nervous anticipation in the air. I see that perhaps some of the men are a bit self-conscious—understandably. Without further delay I face the class and begin.

I introduce myself and present the couples to each other.

"Now," I continue, "I would like to ask each of you why you are here tonight and what you expect from these classes. Would each of you, both husband and wife, tell me your reasons for enrolling?"

The women respond first:

"I want to know exactly what will happen to me and to my baby during labor and delivery."

"I would like to have as little medication as possible. My physician suggested that if I want to help during labor and delivery, if I want to be awake and participate in the birth of my child, then I should attend this course."

"My husband and I want to participate in the birth of our child. A friend of ours attended your classes and told us what wonderful preparation they are."

"I was totally unprepared for the birth of my first child. It was a dreadful experience. This time I want to know what's going on and help myself as well as I can. And I'd like my husband to be with me when I give birth."

And from the men:

"I want to help my wife prepare for childbirth and be with her during labor and delivery."

"My wife's first childbirth was a harrowing experience for both of us. This time I want her to be prepared to help the doctor during labor and have a more pleasant and positive experience. We've heard that this course can do just that."

"Our doctor has said that the exercises, information and respiratory techniques we can learn here are the best possible training and preparation for childbirth."

"Susan asked me to come along tonight. I really don't know what I am supposed to do here. If it were I who had to have the baby, I'd certainly ask the doctor to take care of me and put me to sleep for it. . . ."

"This is an experience we want to share together."

Now we are no longer strangers to each other. We are all here together for the same purpose: to learn about the fabulous engineering feat of giving birth; to gain confidence, a sense of joyous anticipation, a thorough knowledge of how to handle the emotional and physical difficulties—not passively, helpless and unconscious or pacing the hall outside, but as active participants.

WHAT IS PSYCHOPROPHYLACTIC CHILDBIRTH?

Expectant mothers all over the world are preparing in exactly the same way for a conscious, healthy and happy experience. Our technique of preparation is called the psychoprophylactic method of childbirth, or the Lamaze technique. I think you should all know a little about how this technique began and how it spread so rapidly throughout the world.

The late Grantly Dick-Read originated the idea that pain during labor was caused primarily by fear. He wrote in his famous book, *Childbirth Without Fear,* that pain in childbirth could be greatly reduced or even totally eliminated through understanding the process of labor and delivery and through learning to relax properly. Dick-Read felt childbirth is essentially a "normal and physiologic process," and that any pain felt is present because of poor conditioning, the influence of Biblical stories, popular misconceptions, rumors and old wives' tales. Much of this concept has been generally accepted as valid, but we know now that all the education and "cultural conditioning" in the world cannot always provide a childbirth without any pain or discomfort whatsoever.

Dr. Dick-Read called his method "natural childbirth." Unfortunately, over the years the truth in this term has been almost totally obscured by layer upon layer of mysticism. It is thought to be a primitive childbirth, a childbirth completely without help or medication, a kind of endurance test. Dr. Dick-Read's pioneering work was—to a great extent—distorted, and the medical profession, as a result, has become wary of the term and concept of "natural childbirth."

This book presents a series of practical lessons in

5

what we term the psychoprophylactic, or Lamaze, method of childbirth. This method is not a technique of so-called "natural childbirth." On the contrary, it is a technique which is not at all natural, but acquired through concentrated effort and hard work on the part of the expectant mother and her husband. It is a method which provides an analgesic (or lessening of pain) achieved by physical means instead of by drugs or chemical means.

The psychoprophylactic technique originated in Russia, where it was first observed by the late Dr. Fernand Lamaze in 1951. Dr. Lamaze introduced the method to France and other European countries as well as China, Australia, Cuba and South America. In 1959 Marjorie Karmel published her book *Thank You, Dr. Lamaze* here in the United States. It was enormously influential in interesting American physicians and their patients in this new technique. I recommend that each of you read it if you have not already done so.

In 1959 the American Society for Psychoprophylaxis in Obstetrics, Inc., was established. Numerous chapters and affiliates have been formed all over the United States. Now more and more American women and their husbands are preparing for an educated childbirth. American doctors are urging many of their expectant mothers to prepare with this method, and American hospitals are gradually adapting their procedures to allow the active participation of husband and wife in labor and delivery.

What is the theory of the psychoprophylactic method? What does the term psychoprophylaxis mean? It simply means a psychological and physical preparation for childbirth, but you will come to understand it more completely as we work through each lesson together.

HOW DO WE CONTROL PAIN?

Many interesting studies have been made of the nature of pain. We have discovered, for example, that no matter what part of the body provides the source of pain—your foot, knee, abdomen or head—all pain is registered in the cerebral cortex, a part of the brain. It has also been determined that it is not possible to measure the actual *degree* of pain, although its effects, such as changes in blood content, hormonal output, respiration, etc., can be registered.

Experiments have shown that the perception of pain depends on many things that may occur simultaneously with the pain itself. The fact is that we can usually concentrate only on one thing at a time. While we concentrate on one object or sensation, other feelings become peripheral. I'm sure all of you have experiences every day which demonstrate this fact. Let's think of a few examples.

We all know that it is possible to become so engrossed in reading a good book on a train, a subway, or even in a room full of noisy people, that any kind of potential distractions—conversation, whistles, clanging of doors—cannot interrupt our intense concentration. We often hardly notice what is happening around us. We notice the same phenomenon with something that is actually happening within us. Suppose, with a bad headache, you go to the movies and see a really fine film. You may not notice the headache at all while you are watching the picture, but when the film ends, it strikes you with renewed force. What has happened? Simply that your concentration on the film was strong enough to eliminate the perception of pain. When you ceased concentrating, the headache again became the center of your attention.

Another sure way to increase the perception of pain is to overanticipate it. All I have to do is sit down in my dentist's chair and I immediately feel apprehensive and tense. When the dentist asks me to open my mouth so he can look at my teeth I begin to feel pain.

I think most women approach childbirth the same way. They anticipate nothing but pain. "Surely it must hurt. Why are there so many different medications for childbirth if it is not excruciatingly painful?" they ask themselves. And by anticipating and concentrating entirely on the sensation of pain, they leave themselves wide open for real suffering.

No one knows how painful labor actually is. We agree with Dr. Dick-Read that much of the pain in childbirth comes of anxiety and fear, but we do not think that education and "deconditioning" can eliminate it all. We believe that understanding the process of labor and childbirth can alleviate any unnecessary apprehension, and with it *unnecessary* pain. We believe that certain easy exercises can also help prepare the body for a more comfortable labor and delivery. But after all this understanding, education and physical preparation, there is still an undeniable discomfort during childbirth. Our task now is to attack and deal with this residual pain.

Now, if pain in labor were as mild as a headache, I am sure the problem could be solved by installing television sets in every labor room and allowing each expectant mother to watch a fascinating program during delivery. As you can imagine, this technique does not work, but there is nothing wrong with the idea behind it. Our goal throughout these lessons—in addition to understanding what happens during childbirth and learning various exercises to prepare our bodies—will be to recondition ourselves and to create a new center of concentration, thereby causing the awareness of pain to become peripheral. We have found that this is possible not just by looking at an outside object, but by concentrating on a very special activity of our own.

This special activity consists of active and difficult techniques of breathing, which will demand a great amount of concentrated effort. We use different breathing techniques because our breathing is so closely connected with all our activities, whether physical or emotional. Our respiration always automatically synchronizes itself with our activity. When we are asleep, our breathing is very slow. Sitting still, our breathing is also quite slow, but faster than when we are sleeping. When we walk, run, or climb stairs, our breathing changes in rate and intensity. The same changes occur emotionally. Our breathing is slow if we are calm. It speeds up when we are excited or disturbed.

You will learn to change your breathing deliberately during labor, adjusting it to the changing characteristics of the uterine contractions. This will demand an enormous concentrated effort on your part. Not a concentration on pain, but a concentration on your own activity in synchronizing your respiration to the signals that you receive from the uterus. This strenuous activity will create a new center of concentration in the brain, thereby causing the painful sensations during labor to become peripheral, to reduce their intensity. And at the same time, you will learn to relax your body in such a way that you will allow the uterus to work under optimum conditions.

These then are the basic principles of our psychoprophylactic technique of childbirth: education, understanding, preliminary exercises and a technique of special breathing activity and relaxation during labor. I will give you these precision tools to work with. It will be up to you to take these tools and use them as your need demands.

HOW WELL DOES IT WORK?

We are often asked to give statistics about our method. Many physicians want to know whether birth injuries, prematurity, hemorrhaging, etc. can be reduced by using our method. Studies made in France and many other countries show that the psychoprophylactic method does reduce these complications. But there is one important factor that cannot be measured statistically. That is: How does a rewarding experience in childbirth enhance a young couple's relationship with each other? How does the feeling of achievement, of having collaborated in the performance of a difficult job, such as giving birth, affect the husband and wife who have worked hard together toward this goal?

As I have already mentioned, the partner's role is crucial. He must help his wife while she is learning the respiratory techniques. He must see that she is properly relaxed during both practice and actual childbirth. He must help her concentrate on her breathing and signal the length of time between contractions. He must be constantly ready to provide both moral and physical support, not only by his own emotional and physical involvement, but also by the application of specific techniques that we will learn here in class. This can surely be the most joyous and satisfying experience a man and woman can have together.

We women do not give birth very often during our lives. In fact, in our country at this specific period of time, most babies that are born are born by choice and not by chance. This is a very new development, and I'm sure a sociologically and psychologically significant one. I would like to dream and think that a country whose citizens were all desired, might make a wonderful future place for our children to live in. It would be a shame if this great event were to be a traumatic experience, one to be put out of our minds rather than happily remembered. I want to help you make the experience of childbirth a rewarding one which you can perform with dignity and joy, *and* which you and your husband can share together in happy collaboration.

I don't want to make amateur obstetricians out of you. I am sure you have all chosen your doctor or midwife carefully, and that you respect his or her judgment. But I want you to realize that giving birth is really a team effort. The team consists of you and your husband, myself as the teacher, and of course the nurses and your physician. We all have our roles to play.

This brings me to another important point I want to make before we begin our first lesson. I have often been asked the number of successes and failures among my students. I want you to realize that I do not accept the concept of failure in regard to the women I prepare for childbirth. Before we train in our method, we all start off at a point I call minus zero. Every one of you will achieve zero plus, and this will be *your* point of total success. There is no absolute goal, no threshold that all or any of us must reach. You certainly must not feel any kind of guilt or sense of failure if you require some medication, or if you experience discomfort. This is a completely individual thing, depending on the physical nature of your body and its proportions, the size and shape of your baby, and many other factors.

If for any reason medical complications should arise, it is no longer up to you to handle them. Such problems are completely out of your hands, and any decisions of a medical nature lie with your physician. And let us keep in mind that in case mechanical difficulties do occur, your training and active cooperation can frequently help to avoid the use of instruments, or even the necessity of a Caesarean section. Your conscious help and participation can provide invaluable assistance to your physician. You and your doctor will continue to function as a team.

And finally, I think that both of you should visit your doctor together for prenatal examinations. You as women are not having the baby alone. There are two of you creating a family. From the shared beginning through your pregnancy, you are involved together, learning not only to give birth, but how to parent.

LESSON 1

How your body changes during pregnancy;
the importance of good posture;
the three stages of labor: contractions,
delivery of baby, expulsion of placenta

Let's begin this lesson by looking at some pictures (on the following pages) to help you understand the changes that occur in your body during pregnancy.

BODY CHANGES
DURING PREGNANCY

Our first drawing represents the non-pregnant woman. Notice the shape of the uterus. Pay particular attention to the bottleneck opening, which is called the cervix. You can also see the close proximity of the uterus to the bladder, the intestines filling the abdomen, the stomach immediately under the diaphragm, and directly above that, the diaphragm and lungs.

The second drawing shows a pregnant woman, the fetus here about five months old. The uterus is really an extremely elastic, muscular bag. As the baby grows, the uterus expands, moving out of the pelvic cavity into the abdominal cavity, thereby pushing the intestines up and back.

In the third drawing, the fetus is in the ninth month. The uterus now fills the entire abdomen, while the intestines are pushed further up against the stomach and diaphragm, compressing the lungs to a certain degree. This will explain why you are short of breath, why you may occasionally experience heartburn and why your stomach often feels uncomfortable after eating. You can also see how the pressure of the uterus against your bladder is causing all those frequent trips to the bathroom.

Take a closer look at the cervix in drawing number 3. You will observe a small plug at the bottleneck opening. This plug consists of mucus and tiny blood vessels. It prevents bacteria from entering the cervix and causing infection during pregnancy. This plug of mucus is a safety device, and should be reassuring to you. Its presence allows activities such as intercourse, swimming, taking a bath. All these things are considered perfectly safe, unless of course your physician has given you specific instructions to avoid such activities during your pregnancy. Making love during pregnancy is generally considered safe. Perhaps the desire in the woman or in the man may vary in the three trimesters. Obviously you will have to be more inventive and find new positions for intercourse and pleasuring. But don't be afraid to make love. It's virtually impossible to hurt the baby.

As her self-image may suffer somewhat when a woman's figure changes in pregnancy, she may need a great deal of reassurance that she is still desirable. And I can't think of a more delightful way of being reassured than by being loved and making love.

Look at the fourth drawing very carefully. You will notice that the cervix has become shorter, permitting your intestines and stomach more room. The pressure on the bladder has increased. Towards the end of your pregnancy the baby is likely to drop, settling into the pelvic cavity. This is not a sudden drop, but gradual. At this point, you will notice that, although you can breathe more easily, there is increased pressure on your bladder and thighs.

Perhaps well-meaning people will tell you how "low" you carry, and overwhelm you with tales of what this might mean. Take no notice of their well-meant advice, but rather ask your doctor if you are in doubt about any symptom or discomfort. Your doctor will tell you now that the head of your baby has become "engaged." What does this mean? It's really quite simple: the head has entered the pelvis, a cavity composed of the sacrum, the iliac bone, and the symphysis pubis. The engagement of the baby's head is an encouraging sign.

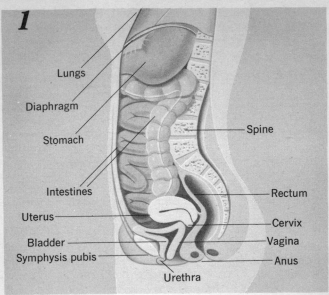

1

Lungs

Diaphragm

Stomach

Intestines

Uterus

Bladder

Symphysis pubis

Spine

Rectum

Cervix

Vagina

Anus

Urethra

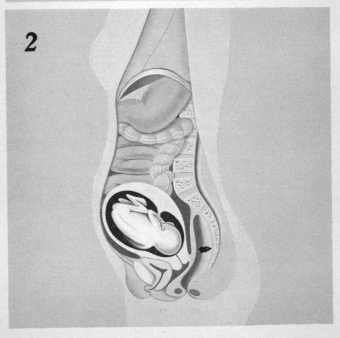

2

1. This illustration shows the position of the uterus in a non-pregnant woman and its relation to the other organs

2. At five months the baby has entered the abdominal cavity, exerting some pressure against the diaphragm and lungs

3. In ninth month the baby fills nearly the entire abdomen but nonetheless internal organs continue to function well

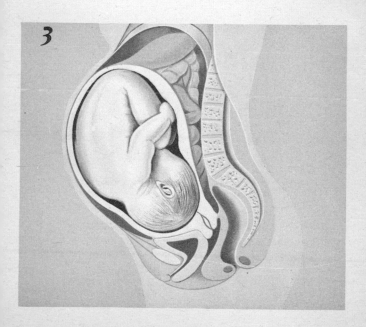

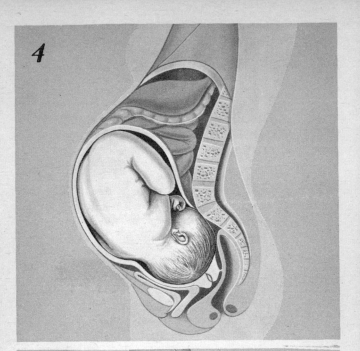

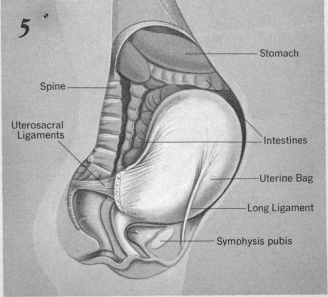

Stomach

Spine

Uterosacral
Ligaments

Intestines

Uterine Bag

Long Ligament

Symphysis pubis

4. At the end of the ninth month the baby's head has become engaged, wedged now between pubic bone and sacrum

5. This shows the baby as it is contained in the uterine bag, which is supported by ligaments at the sides and the back

You now know that you are getting closer to labor. This may happen as long as three weeks before your due date, or it may happen only a few days before you go into labor. Occasionally the head will engage only when you are already in labor.

The fifth drawing shows the entire uterine bag. This bag is supported by ligaments, which act like columns supporting a building. There are two long ligaments, one on each side, and two short ones attached to the lower part of your spine. You may occasionally feel a sharp pain in your groin when you stretch suddenly, cough or sneeze. This picture shows you that such an occasional sudden pain is caused by stretching the long ligaments. The pain is of no consequence, and I hope you will be better able to put up with this occasional discomfort now that you realize what causes it.

IMPORTANCE OF GOOD POSTURE

The ligaments attached to your lower spine may cause backache during pregnancy. Backache in pregnancy is a frequent occurrence. Unfortunately we often increase the normal strain on our back by poor posture. It is so easy for us to take the line of least resistance when carrying a heavy baby. By letting the abdomen hang and leaning back slightly we weaken our abdominal muscles, simply by not using them. We may also strain the back muscles by overextending them. It is of the utmost importance that we learn to use our bodies correctly during pregnancy.

When standing we must always remember that the crown of our head is the highest part of the body. If you raise your head as indicated in the next pictures you find that the rest of your body aligns itself. There is no need to tuck in your bottom or your abdominal muscles. This will naturally occur if you thus raise your head.

You will find that good posture will enable you to walk more gracefully, putting far less strain on your abdominal and back muscles. And believe it or not, you will find that good posture will ease the pressure on your bladder. I suggest that your husband remind you now and then to "stretch up."

Good posture will also prevent fatigue. It is normal for you to tire more easily when you are pregnant, but don't let your tiredness accumulate. Rest during the day, if only for ten minutes at a time. Sit down, or better still, lie down with your legs raised. You will soon feel your energy coming back and be able to get through a long day with greater ease.

Here is another exercise which will help you to strengthen the pelvic floor, make it more elastic, and make you more aware of your pelvic floor muscles, which you'll have to relax when you have to push your baby out. The exercise is called the "Kegel exercise," after the late Dr. Kegel, who described and used the exercise in the treatment of incontinence and poor pelvic muscle tone.

I will teach you now to exercise your pubio-coccygeal muscle, which is the muscle band leading from near the pubic bone to near the coccyx. This muscle is shaped like a figure of eight, it surrounds your sphincters and passages, and its most important function is to support the bladder, the vagina and uterus, and the rectum.

Sit comfortably, legs slightly apart; lean forward a

little. Now tighten your front passage as if to stop yourself from urinating. Then squeeze your vagina, and finally tighten your back passage as if you were preventing a bowel movement. Hold it—one—two—three —four—five—six—and release. Think "release" and you will find that you can relax even more. Always connect your body movements with your mind. If you think the movement, you will find that you can perform the exercise much more thoroughly.

Repeat this Kegel exercise at least 20–30 times a day. You can do it in a standing, sitting or lying position; while driving your car, in the subway or bus, at boring parties or during TV commercials. Nobody will ever notice you are doing it. However, you will soon notice that you are carrying your baby better, there will be less pressure on your thighs, and as a special bonus, you and your partner will find that love making is even more fun when you have the ability to contract and relax your vaginal muscles easily.

Exercising your pelvic floor muscles will improve the muscle tone and increase the elasticity of your perineum—the area between the anus and the vulva—so that it will stretch easily when your baby descends. Frequent use of these muscles will also make you conscious of their position and function, and will enable you to help the smooth expulsion of your baby through conscious neuromuscular control, just as the "concentration-relaxation" exercises trained you to develop relaxation and control over your arms, legs and facial muscles.

Practice this exercise diligently from now until you give birth. It is also one of the most important exercises to do shortly *after* you've given birth. Once you have delivered the baby and are back in your room, start contracting your pelvic floor. Or even on the delivery table. You will probably feel sore and numb in your pelvic area. The stitches from your episiotomy may feel irritated. You may be afraid to urinate or have a bowel movement. By using your Kegel exercises there

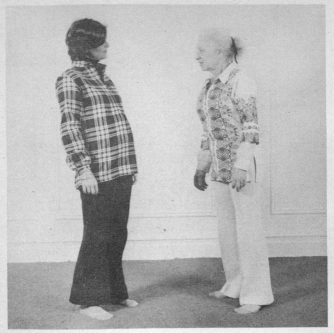

*Gail demonstrates a very poor posture—
one that will give her a backache and will
weaken her abdominal muscles*

and then, you can speed up the healing process of the episiotomy and begin a much more comfortable post-partum (after delivery) period.

I would like every woman to practice this pelvic-floor exercise for the rest of her life in order to retain good muscle tone. This may prevent weakness or even a prolapse in later life.

Now let us look at the following pictures so that we may see the actual process of labor. In the illustration on page 26 you see a baby ready to be born. The mother is lying on her back. You will recognize the spine, the

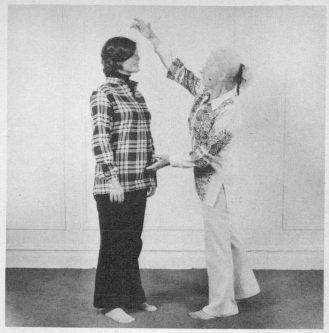

*Lifting the top of the head correctly aligns
the body, supports the baby and helps
reduce pressure on the bladder*

anus, the vagina, the urinary opening or urethra, the
uterus with its bottleneck cervix (which in this picture
has lost its plug) and of course the baby, which is facing the mother's hip.

THE FIRST
STAGE OF LABOR

Labor is divided into three stages. During the first
stage, the uterus begins to contract involuntarily—that

is, entirely on its own—thereby pulling on the cervix. The cervix becomes soft, thins out and flattens. This is called the *effacement* of the cervix. In the majority of women, the effacement starts towards the end of pregnancy, as early as two to three weeks before the birth of the baby. You may have already felt an occasional tightening in your abdomen. These tightenings are contractions of the uterus and are entirely painless. These preliminary contractions are called Braxton-Hicks contractions. They are named after an Englishman, Mr. Braxton-Hicks, who was the first to describe them in medical literature. Once labor proper begins, you will feel the uterine contractions more distinctly. These new, stronger contractions will cause the cervix to dilate.

The opening of the cervix can be compared to the neck of a very tight turtleneck sweater. Imagine yourself trying to put the sweater on: You pull it and stretch it until you have finally opened it far enough for you to push your head through. Thus the uterus has to pull on the cervix and stretch it with each contraction until it has opened to the widest diameter of the baby's head. Only then can you start to push your baby out. We say that the first stage of labor has ended when the cervix has opened fully to "5 fingers" or "10 centimeters."

I would like you to remember both these terms for the dilation of the cervix. Your doctor will examine you internally during labor and let you know how far along you are in precisely this language. He'll say you are "3 fingers" or "7 centimeters" open. I feel that communication between you and your physician is of the utmost importance before and during your labor. It is therefore essential for you to be acquainted with this terminology. Thus you can be fully aware of all the signposts on your road through labor to delivery.

THE SECOND
STAGE OF LABOR

The door is now open. The second stage of labor is the expulsion of the baby. The uterus now works like a piston expelling the baby. Your lungs, diaphragm and strong abdominal muscles will provide the necessary power for this piston. You will see, in the picture on page 28, that the baby has rotated now and that the symphysis pubis acts as a pivotal point or fulcrum for the baby. The baby now faces the mother's spine and its head is at an angle. As the head gradually pushes through the vagina or birth canal the crown appears at the vulva or outlet of the vagina. At this point the doctor will talk of the "crowning" of the baby's head. The head now emerges, and you will see from the next illustrations that it is being rotated once again (this time externally, with the help of the doctor), to aid the expulsion of the shoulders. Once the shoulders have been delivered, the rest of the baby's body will slip out easily. The birth of the baby is the end of the second stage of labor.

A moment before you deliver the baby's head your doctor may make a small incision, called the "episiotomy," in the mouth of the vagina. This minor surgical procedure is performed to avoid possible tearing of your tissue as the baby's head is delivered. Your physician will decide whether or not an episiotomy is necessary. It is quite commonly done in America, since a small, neat incision can be easily repaired, and heals quickly. A tear with a ragged edge may create difficulties. The incision is frequently done with a local anesthetic.

It is important for you to realize that an episiotomy does not in any way interfere with your desire and ability to use the psychoprophylactic method of childbirth. In fact it is good to remember once again that

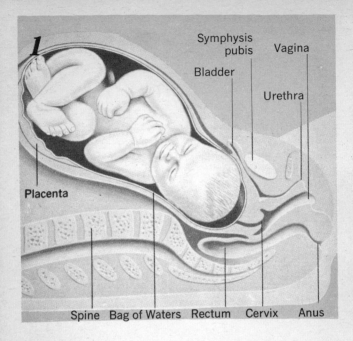

1

Symphysis
pubis

Vagina

Bladder

Urethra

Placenta

Spine   Bag of Waters   Rectum   Cervix   Anus

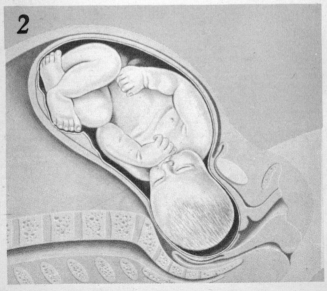

2

1. This baby is ready to be born: the mother is lying on her back, her baby facing her right hip; the cervix is still thick and long; preliminary contractions have not yet occurred

2. Here begins the first stage of labor: contractions have started; the baby has begun to move down and the cervix becomes shorter and flatter in the process called effacement

3. Baby rotates slightly as contractions during the first stage of labor continue. The cervix dilates; here it has opened about halfway, which is termed 2½ fingers or 5 centimeters

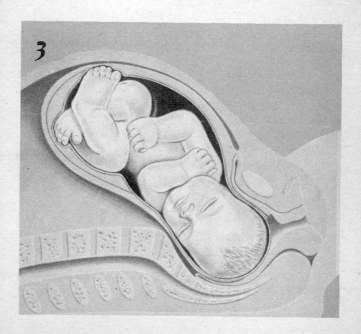

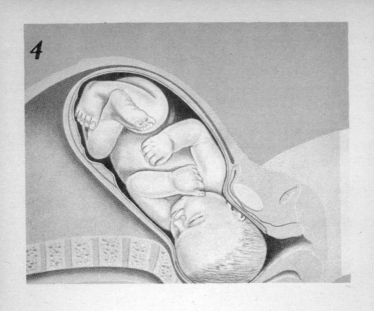

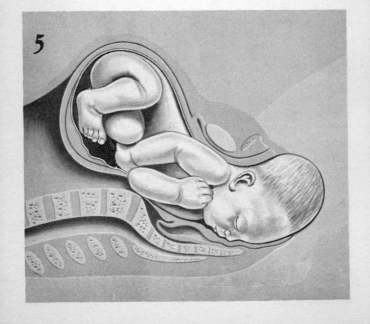

4. At the end of the first stage of labor, cervix is fully dilated (5 fingers or 10 centimeters); the baby's head is entering the stretched vagina and putting pressure upon the rectum

5. During second stage of labor, the baby faces the mother's spine, flexing and extending its soft head to pivot around the pubic bone as it is pushed on through the birth canal

6. The head rotates once again on delivery to allow the shoulders and arms to emerge; the rest of the body slips out easily; expulsion is completed and the baby is born

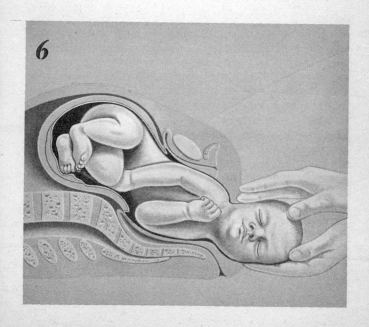

your labor and delivery will involve teamwork between you and your husband and between you and your physician. The performance or nonperformance of an episiotomy will be entirely your doctor's responsibility, though you should discuss your ideas and feelings about this process with your doctor, and you should know what you can do to acquire good control of your pelvic floor muscles to help yourself and the doctor. Don't forget to practice these exercises at least 20–30 times a day.

THE THIRD
STAGE OF LABOR

The third stage of labor is the expulsion of the afterbirth or "placenta." Once the baby has been born, the doctor will clamp and cut the umbilical cord. This procedure does not hurt either you or your baby. A few minutes after the birth of your child your uterus will contract again and your doctor will ask you to push once more to expel the placenta. He will generally help you by exerting pressure on your abdomen. The expulsion of the placenta is generally very fast, taking only a few minutes.

This has been our first class. For the next session I would like you to wear shorts, tights, slacks or any comfortable garment that will allow you to perform our exercises easily. We will continue to look at these pictures and discuss the process of labor in more detail. I will never teach an exercise by itself, but will always explain—with the help of these pictures—why we perform certain exercises during each phase of labor.

LESSON 2

Learning to relax and conserve your
energy through neuromuscular control
exercises; simple but basic exercises
to prepare your body for childbirth

This lesson will be a more active one for you and your husband. We are going to do exercises today, which I divide into two groups:

1. Neuromuscular control exercises, which I also call Concentration-Relaxation exercises.
2. Body-building or limbering-up, exercises.

One of the primary aims during labor must be the conservation of energy. You should never exert more energy than is actually needed for efficient performance during this period. By conserving energy you will avoid unnecessary fatigue. If you are tense, if you thrash around or dig your fingernails into the mattress (or your partner's arm), you are wasting energy.

NEUROMUSCULAR CONTROL EXERCISES

Neuromuscular control exercises are extremely important. You must remember that the uterus will be working hard during labor. That part of your body will be extremely active. Your task will be to allow it to work freely while you keep the rest of your body deliberately relaxed. These exercises will help you to develop muscle control, to isolate muscle groups, and at the same time make you aware of which muscle groups are in use and which are at rest.

These exercises will have to be practiced with your partner. Not only is it impossible for you to check on your own relaxation, but I want your partner to give the commands, which I will demonstrate. I also want him to check on your tension and relaxation. In this way you will learn to react to your partner's signals instantly, and he will learn to recognize any tensions in your body. You will be involved in labor and may not notice that while trying to control the uterine contractions, you have tensed your legs or arms or face. Your partner, however, will see these tensions immediately, and you will be able to cooperate and relax whenever he gives the signal. I think the great advantage of your working together is that since you have shared your lives for some time, you know each other very well, and are therefore much more aware of each other's tensions and difficulties than a strange nurse or doctor could ever be. And this intimate knowledge can be used in working together in labor and correcting tensions. I am often sure that I can tell what kind of day my husband has had when he comes home, even before he has said a word. It's his facial expression, perhaps, or the way he holds his shoulders. I'm not even sure what it is. Try it sometime with your partner. Watch him or her, and soon you'll be able to spot tensions and weak points. This will make it easier to react to each other's signals.

This will require considerable discipline from both of you. Your partner's commands have to be as disciplined as your reaction. By developing this kind of teamwork, it will be easy for you to react to his signals, even under stress.

Lie on the floor, on your back, a pillow under your head and another pillow or bolster under your knees. Begin by taking a very deep and relaxing inhalation-exhalation. I call such a deep relaxing breath "a cleansing breath." From now on, when I speak of a "cleansing breath," you will know that I want you to take a deep breath, then exhale and relax your whole body. Your partner should now check your relaxation. Let him gently lift your arm by holding your wrist in his hand and feeling the whole weight of your arm and shoulder. Let your arm bend at the elbow so that every joint is relaxed. Once your partner feels the weight of your arm, he can then try to move your arm freely from side to side to check on your absolute relaxation. When he lets go of your arm, it should drop heavily to the floor. Let him try your other arm. To check the relaxation of your legs, your partner must place his hands under your knees and gently lift them a little off the pillow. Your heels should remain on the floor. If your leg is tense, he will not be able to bend your knee easily and he should therefore give the command, "Relax."

Once your partner is satisfied that you are relaxed, he should give the following command: "Contract your right arm." You will then tense your arm, shoulder, elbow, fist, and raise your arm, holding it straight before you a few inches off the floor. Your partner should check on the tension in your right arm, then check on the complete relaxation of your left arm and both legs —while you are still holding up your right arm. The next command is: "Release your arm," and your arm should fall absolutely relaxed to the floor.

Command: "Contract your left arm." Tense the arm, shoulder, elbow, fist, and raise your left arm, holding it straight before you, a few inches off the floor. Again your partner should check first on the tension in your left arm and then, while the left arm is tense, he must check on the relaxation of your right arm and both your legs. Next command: "Release your left arm."

Command: "Contract your right leg." Stiffen your thigh, hold the leg straight and flex your foot. You don't have to raise your leg. While you are holding your leg stiff, your partner should check first on the tension of the right leg, then on the relaxation of your left leg and both arms, checking your shoulders and face at the same time. Command: "Release your leg."

Command: "Contract right arm, right leg." Again your partner will check on your tension on the right side and your release of muscles on your left. "Release."

Command: "Contract left arm, left leg." Be sure to stiffen your leg well and to flex your foot in order to

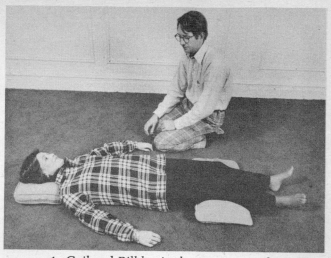

1. Gail and Bill begin the neuromuscular control exercises. Note complete relaxation, good support under head, knees.

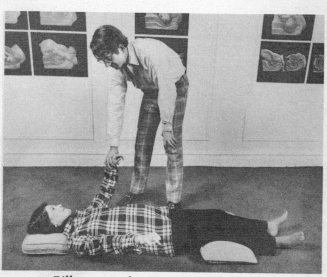

2. Bill commands: "Contract right arm", as Gail responds he checks carefully to make sure that her left arm is relaxed

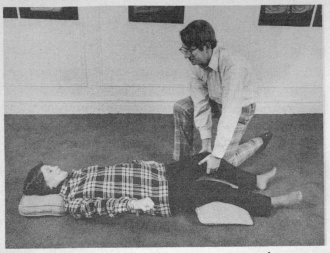

3. While Gail's right arm is contracted,
Bill checks on the relaxation of her legs
by lifting her knees from the pillow

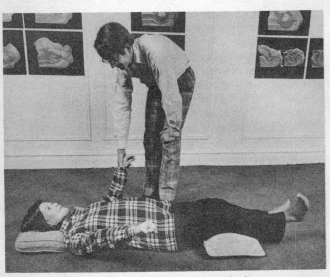

4. "Contract right arm and right leg."
Again Bill must make sure that both her
left arm and left leg remain relaxed

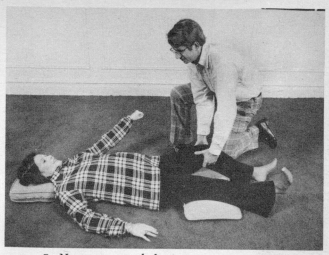

5. Now commands become more complex as Gail must contract her opposing arms and legs while Bill checks carefully

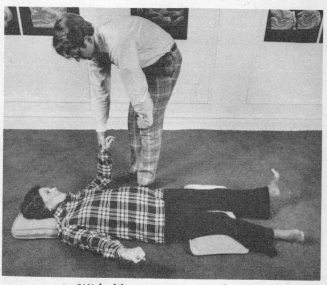

6. With diligent practice and Bill's cooperation, Gail learns to concentrate and relax in automatic response to command

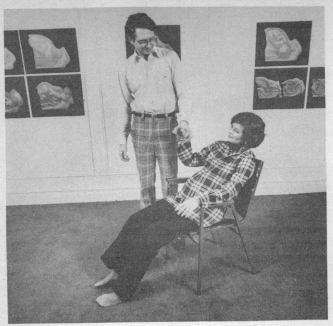

7. *Gail relaxes in an alternate position: sitting.*
Bill checks the relaxation of her right arm

tense the calf muscles. Your partner will check your tension and relaxation. "Release."

Command: "Contract your right arm, left leg." Your partner will check and give the command: "Release."

Command: "Contract your left leg, arm, right leg." Your partner will check and release.

You will soon realize how very difficult it is to work with one part of your body while keeping the rest of your body relaxed. It will demand your absolute concentration and special attention. You will discover that only with continued and repeated practice will you be able to isolate muscle groups and automatically follow your partner's signals. You should practice these exercises at least once a day. Let me point out once again that the purpose of these exercises is to make you aware of your body, to establish a source of teamwork between you and your partner and to enable you to be economical with all energy expended during labor. If lying down is difficult for you, the exercise can be easily performed in a comfortable chair. You realize, of course, that you won't tense and lift an arm in labor, or tense a leg. This exercise is a training for labor, to make you become aware of your body and thus able to separate muscle groups, relaxing part of your body as other parts are working.

BODY-BUILDING EXERCISES

I think we all tend to slow down considerably during pregnancy, partly because of the added weight we have to carry, partly because of our own anxiety that we might somehow injure the baby when we stretch, bend or simply move around. So many people shower us with well-meant advice not to do this, that, or the other. I am sure you have been told by someone not to reach or raise your arms above your head, not to cross your legs, etc. If we really followed all this well-intended counsel, we could hardly move at all.

It is perfectly safe to lead a normal life and to move about as much as you have always done, as long as it does not hurt and you don't get too tired. I always like to quote Dr. Alan Guttmacher here. He told us once that as a young obstetrician he used to forbid his patients to play tennis, though he allowed every other sport. In discussing this with a colleague, the colleague said, "Strange, I forbid my patients to do swimming and allow them to do anything else!" They realized that they were both discouraging the particular sport they themselves didn't like or were poor at.

The limbering-up exercises I will show you are meant to make you feel better *now*. They will strengthen your back and abdominal muscles so you can carry the additional weight of the baby with comparative

EXERCISE 1

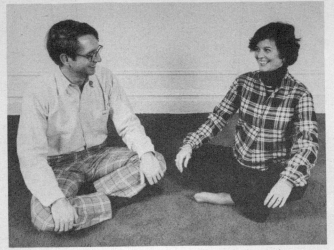

Bill and Gail assume a basic position, sitting tailor-fashion; this helps to stretch the pelvis and the muscles of the thigh

ease. They will help you to spread your legs far apart, which will be most useful for you when you have to push out your baby. Some of the exercises will improve the tone of your pelvic-floor muscles.

For the following exercises you do not need a pillow under your head or knees. And don't practice any of these exercises on your bed, even if you think your mattress is very hard. The hardest mattress is still too soft. You need firm support. Use the floor, covered by a rug or blanket.

Exercise 1: Sit cross-legged (tailor fashion) on the floor, back relaxed and slightly rounded. Use this sitting position as much as possible from now on. It will help to strengthen your pelvic-floor muscles and stretch your thigh muscles. We rarely sit in this position any more, with all our comfortable upholstered chairs and couches. I suggest you do this in the evenings while

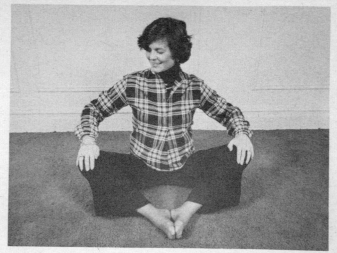

To stretch her muscles more, Gail puts
the soles of her feet together and
exerts slight pressure upon her knees

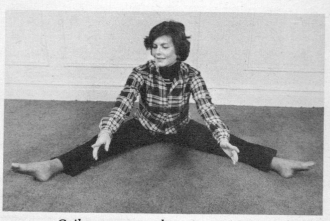

Gail assumes an alternate position to
stretch her pelvis and her thighs

you read, sew, watch television or play chess with your husband. When you get tired of sitting like this, stretch your legs for a while, shake them out, then resume the position.

Exercise 2: Sit on the floor and put the soles of your feet together, then pull your feet as close to your body as possible. Put your hands on your thighs and press them gently down. You will feel the muscles pull on the inside of your thighs. For those of you who have very long ligaments, this exercise may be very easy. Your thighs will practically touch the floor with little effort. If so, try the following exercise: Sit on the floor, stretch your legs well apart and turn your knees out. Then lean your body forward, and you will feel a good pull in your thighs.

Exercise 3: Lie on your back, arms at your sides. Take a deep, cleansing breath. Now raise your right leg up slowly, pointing your toes, breathing in slowly through your nose. Be sure to keep both knees straight. Then flex your foot, lower your leg slowly to the ground and at the same time exhale through your mouth and lips. Repeat with your left leg. Take care to synchronize your breathing with the raising and lowering of your leg, to point your toes as you go up, and to flex your foot as you go down, keeping both legs straight at all times. Repeat this exercise five times for each leg.

Exercise 4: Lie on your back, stretching your arms at right angles from your body. Take a deep cleansing breath. Then raise your right leg, pointing your toes and inhaling through your nose. Follow this by flexing your foot, and lower your leg to the right side as far as is comfortable as you breathe out through your mouth. Then point your toes, inhale through your nose and raise your leg; flex your foot and lower your leg to the floor, as you breathe out through your mouth. Repeat this with the left leg. See to it that the hip opposite the moving leg remains flat on the floor. Work on this exercise so that you can do it at least three times with each leg.

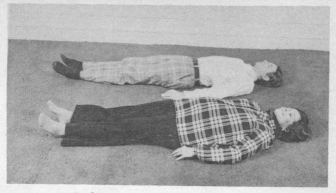

1. To begin this body-building exercise, Gail and Bill lie flat on a hard floor with no support, inhaling and exhaling deeply

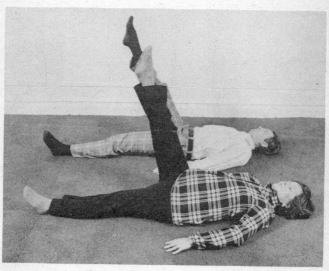

2. As Gail and Bill inhale through their nose, they raise their right legs slowly, keeping their knees straight and toes pointed

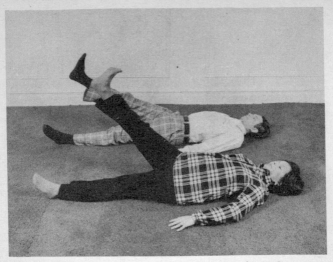

3. Gail and Bill flex feet, exhale through their lips and lower legs slowly, synchronizing their breathing and their movements

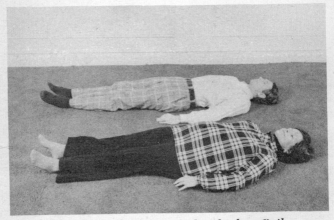

4. The exercise is completed when Gail and Bill have raised each leg five times and take a deep inhalation-exhalation to relax

VARIATION
OF EXERCISE 3

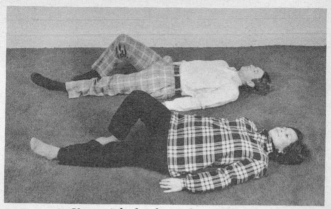

1. Keep right leg bent, foot resting on
the door, inhaling and exhaling deeply

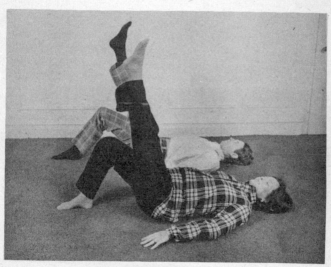

2. Stretch left leg up, pointing
the toes and inhaling comfortably

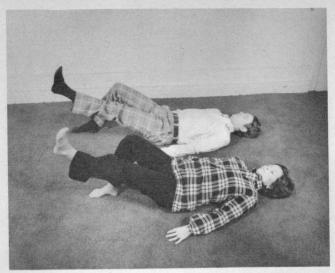

3. Flex foot and lower leg slowly as you exhale

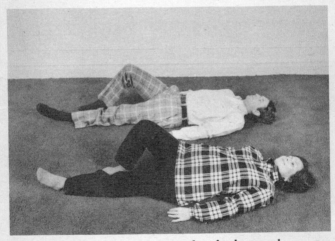

4. The exercise is completed when each leg has been raised five times and a deep inhalation-exhalation taken to relax

EXERCISE 4

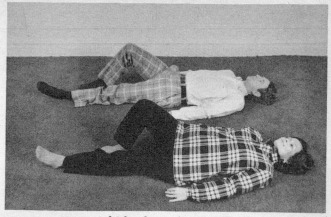

1. Keep right leg bent, foot resting on the floor, inhaling and exhaling deeply

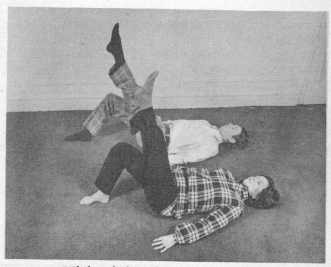

2. While inhaling through nose, raise leg as high as you can, pointing your toes

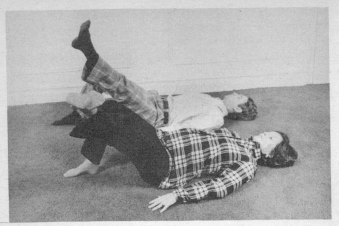

3. At point of highest elevation flex your foot and lower your leg slowly outward toward the arm of the same side

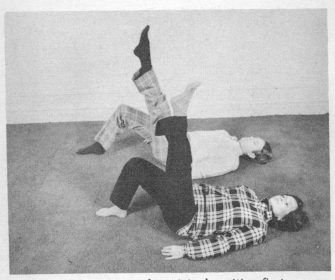

4. To return to the original position first point your toes, raise your leg up again, and inhale through your nose

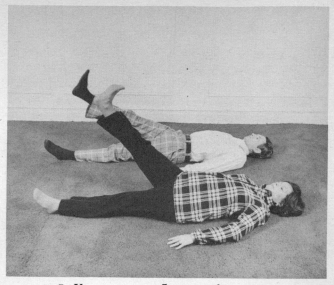

5. You must now flex your foot again;
exhale slowly through your mouth while
gradually lowering your leg to the floor

Exercise 5: This is my favorite. It strengthens the back
as well as the abdominal muscles. It is a good exercise
whether you are pregnant or not. Have your husband
do it as well, particularly if he often feels tired or his
back is bothering him.

Again lie on your back and bend your knees so that
your feet are firmly on the ground. Press your entire
back, including your shoulders, firmly against the floor,
pulling in the lower abdominal muscles at the same
time and letting your buttocks lift very slightly off the
floor. Then release. This exercise should be done with
controlled breathing. Start by breathing in, then exhale
through your mouth slowly and, as you exhale, press
your back against the floor, contracting your abdominal
muscles. Breathe in as you release your back and abdomen. You will find that you can flatten your back

EXERCISE 5

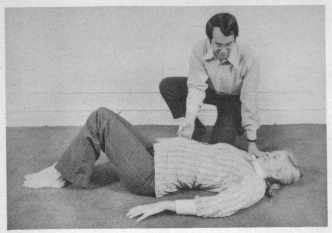

1. Barbara does the important back exercise on the floor with bent knees, inhaling slowly and keeping her back relaxed

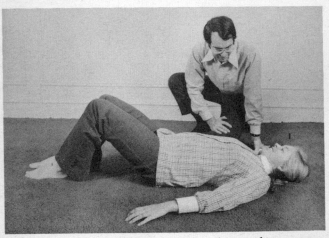

2. Now she exhales slowly, flattens her shoulders and back against the hard floor, contracts her abdominal muscles, while Tom checks that she flattens her back completely against the floor

EXERCISE 6

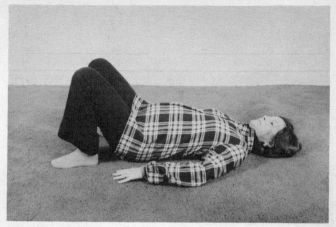

1. Lie on your back, knees and feet
separated, feet firmly on the ground

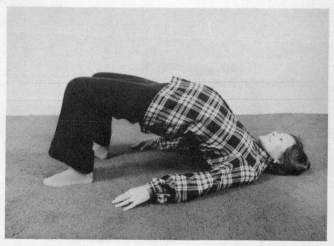

2. Raise your buttocks off the floor, hips
raised toward the ceiling, as you breathe in

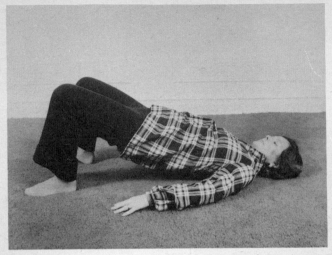

*3. Lower your back slowly, vertebra
by vertebra, as you exhale*

much more effectively if you exhale when doing it. Be
sure to use correct breathing techniques: exhale when
you flatten yourself: inhale when you release your back.
Exercise 6: Lie on your back and bend your knees, feet
firmly on the ground. This time, separate your feet and
bring your heels as close to your buttocks as possible.
Now breathe in and raise your buttocks and back off
the floor—push your hips toward the ceiling. Then as
you exhale slowly, lower your back, vertebra by vertebra, like a "string of pearls," bit by bit. Keep your
hips up till the end, then slowly lower them and rest.
Repeat this exercise three times.
Exercise 7: Sit cross-legged and stretch your arms up
high. Look at your fingertips and pull yourself out of
your ribs. If you really look at your fingertips, you can
stretch another half-inch. Now relax.

EXERCISE 7

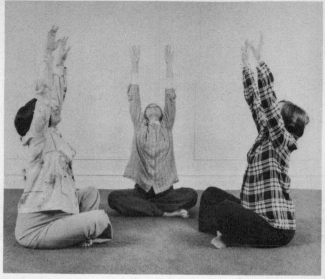

1. *Felice, Barbara and Gail stretch spinal columns, looking up at their finger-tips*

We will start with our third group of exercises, respiration exercises, in the next lesson. Be sure to practice daily with your partner, so that he can supervise and correct you, and so that both of you can understand the purpose of our first two groups of exercises.

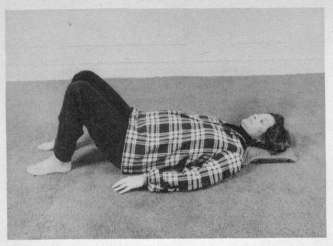

1. During pregnancy, be sure to rise
from a lying position in a manner that
will not strain your abdominal muscles

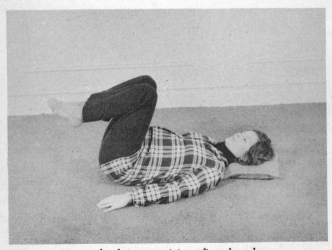

2. From the lying position, first bend your
legs and knees up, still supporting
yourself with both hands at your sides

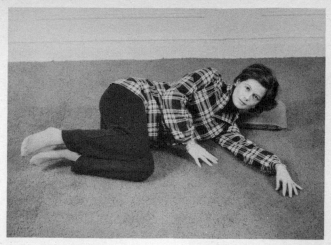

3. Keeping your legs parallel, roll over to one side so that your weight rests on one hip, supported by both hands

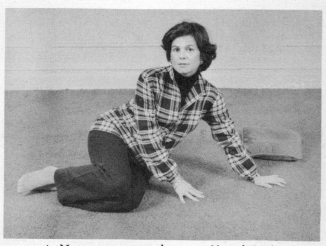

4. Now you can push yourself with both hands to a sitting position from which it will be easy for you to stand up

LESSON 3

Three phases of uterine contractions:
latent, accelerated, transitional;
our first breathing technique; partner's
role during practice at home

It is always important to review the material covered in our previous lesson. These reviews are an essential aspect of your training. Not that I don't trust you to practice diligently, but it is imperative to see how proficient you have become, and to correct a few things that you may have misunderstood. Therefore bear with me when I encourage you to repeat and repeat the exercises. This is the discipline of the Lamaze technique. You will have to learn to channel your energy correctly for your labor, and I will help you do so.

Let us review the neuromuscular control exercises. Do you remember what these are for? Do we actually tense one arm or leg in labor? Certainly not. These exercises will teach you to relax part of your body while the rest is working, and they will also help to establish teamwork between you and your partner. Lie comfortably on the floor, a pillow under your head, a bolster under your knees. Take a deep "cleansing breath" and relax. Let your partner check your relaxation before he gives the commands.

Then: Contract right arm. Release. Contract left arm (partner should check thoroughly). Release. Contract right arm and right leg (partner checks). Release. Contract left arm and left leg (partner checks). Release. Contract right arm and left leg (partner checks). Release. Contract left arm and right leg (partner checks). Release.

I hope you will notice how much you have improved in one week. It should be much easier for you to isolate muscle groups and to follow your partner's commands. Some of you will learn faster than others, but in a relatively short time you will have learned this difficult body control. Remember also that it is really a good idea to have this control whether you are pregnant or not.

Now let us review the body-building exercises. These can be done without your partner's help. Take the pillows away and sit on the floor cross-legged. Then put the soles of your feet together, your hands on your thighs, and press your thighs gently down.

Next lie on your back, arms at your sides. Take a deep cleansing breath. Raise your right leg slowly, pointing your toes. Breathe in slowly through your nose as you raise your leg. Flex your foot, lower your leg, keep your knee straight, and breathe out slowly through your mouth. Repeat with your left leg. Repeat this exercise five times for each leg, or the variation to this exercise (p. 45).

Lie on your back on the floor. Extend your arms at right angles to your sides. Inhale and exhale deeply. Bend left leg. While inhaling through your nose, raise right leg up as far as you can, pointing your toes, keeping your knee straight. Then lower your leg gently to the right as far as is comfortable, flexing your foot and exhaling through your mouth. Then inhaling again, raise your leg to upright position, while pointing your toes. Finally, exhale slowly and lower your leg again to its original position, flexing your foot. Inhale and exhale deeply. Repeat this series with your left leg. Do this exercise at least three times with each leg.

Lie on your back, bend your knees and keep your feet firmly on the floor. Press your back hard against the floor, straightening it right to your shoulders, tightening your lower abdominal muscles at the same time. Then release your back. Do not forget to exhale when you flatten your back, and inhale when you release your back.

Lie on your back, bend your knees, feet firmly on the floor, heels close to your buttocks. Inhale and slowly raise your back off the floor, hips against the ceiling, then exhale slowly as you lower your back vertebra by vertebra and rest your back.

Here is the last exercise: the spinal stretch. Sit cross-legged, bend your arms to your shoulders, then stretch them well into the air. Look at your fingertips, stretch a little more, and a little more, and a little more. Then relax and breathe deeply. You will find it feels wonderful to be able to stretch, and you can rest assured that it will not do you or the baby any harm whatsoever.

If any of you have been to physical fitness or dance classes, you will probably be able to think of other suitable exercises. Be sure, however, never to raise or lower both legs at the same time when you are lying flat on your back.

THE THREE PHASES OF THE FIRST STAGE OF LABOR

I want you to look once again at the pictures and drawings showing the first stage of labor. You will remember that the first stage of labor consists of the effacement—or thinning out and flattening—of the cervix, and its dilation to 5 fingers or 10 centimeters.

We divide the first stage of labor into three parts or phases.

Part One is the *latent* or *preliminary* phase of labor, during which the cervix effaces fully and dilates to about 1½ fingers or 3 centimeters.

Part Two is the dilation of the cervix from about 1½ fingers or 3 centimeters to approximately 4 fingers or 8 centimeters. This phase is called the *accelerated,* or active phase of labor.

Part Three is the dilation of the cervix from 4 fingers to full dilation or 5 fingers or, in centimeters, from 8 to 10. This phase is called the *transition* phase.

The uterine contractions change their character in the three phases of the first stage of labor. The uterus, like any other muscle in our body, contracts and relaxes. This is the nature of muscle. Stretch your arm out, then bend it slowly. In doing this, you have used a muscle—that is, you have contracted the biceps.

When you straighten your arm again you release the tension in the biceps. Suppose you were to draw a diagram of a muscular contraction, it would look like a curve, or a wave pattern.

Look at the diagrams on page 62, which will show you the changes in the waves that occur during the three phases of the first stage of labor. I like to compare these waves to those at the oceanside. There are many people, and you may be among them, who can surf-ride very well, meeting each wave with confidence and riding with it and through it. And then there are people like myself: I don't know how to cope with these waves. Should I face them? Should my back be turned towards them? And before I have managed to make up my mind, the wave has hit me, thrown me over. I scrape my knees, get water in my mouth and nose and scramble out exhausted, telling myself not to try again until the next summer.

I think one can compare the trained or untrained woman in labor to the person who has learned or who has not learned to ride the waves at the beach.

A few years ago, though, a friend showed me how to manage the waves when we were swimming together, and though I never became an expert at it, I could manage to ride, if not most, at least many of the waves—and I felt very good about it. Even if I missed one, I was confident that I could cope with the next one. And so it is in labor: you probably won't catch every wave; you'll goof occasionally, but you will stay on top of most of them, and you will say as one of my students said, "it actually got easier and easier the more labor progressed, because I got better and better." Another of my students told me, "The fact that I could participate in the birth of my child and knew what to do and actively give birth, was the greatest ego trip I've ever had in my life!"

In the *preliminary* or *latent phase* of labor (1) the waves are gentle and shallow. One wave may last from 30 to 60 seconds, and the intervals of rest may vary

3 PHASES OF
FIRST STAGE OF LABOR

1

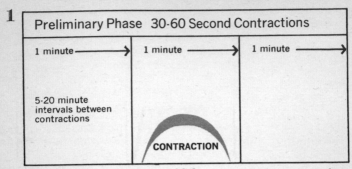

Preliminary Phase   30-60 Second Contractions

1 minute →   1 minute →   1 minute →

5-20 minute intervals between contractions

CONTRACTION

During this early phase of labor, contractions occur in the form of mild waves that come at irregular intervals

2

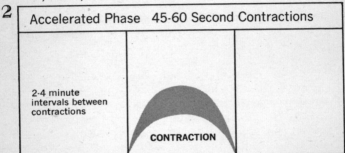

Accelerated Phase   45-60 Second Contractions

2-4 minute intervals between contractions

CONTRACTION

The accelerated phase is the longest and most active period of labor. Waves become higher and last longer

3

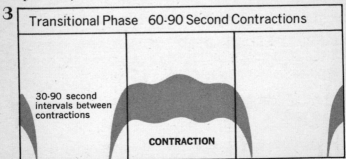

Transitional Phase   60-90 Second Contractions

30-90 second intervals between contractions

CONTRACTION

This phase is the most intense and the shortest phase of the first stage of labor. Waves are erratic and sharp

BREATHING EXERCISES FOR FIRST STAGE OF LABOR

1

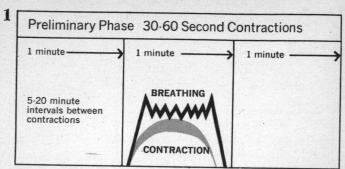

Begin wave with cleansing breath, follow with 6-9 chest inhalation-exhalations, conclude with cleansing breath

2

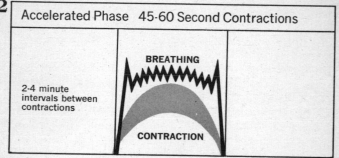

Take cleansing breath; accelerate breathing as wave rises, decelerate as it subsides; finish with a cleansing breath

3

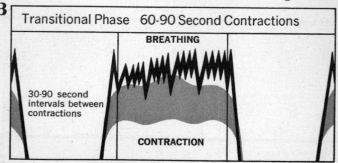

Take cleansing breath; continue pattern of 4-6 breaths, then a short blowing out; take a final cleansing breath

from 5 to 20 minutes. This first phase of labor, where the contractions are mild, lasts quite a long time. A study of the labor of many women has shown that the average time may be about 8 to 9 hours. For most of this period you will probably be at home, and you won't even need any breathing control for a great part of this phase.

If you are one of those very rare women who do have extremely easy and fast labors, you may not need every step of our training. But I would much rather have you prepare yourself for the average: a normal, lengthy labor. Should labor be faster than you anticipated, you will find that you are prepared to cope. For second or third babies, the average time limits for the three phases of the first stage of labor will be about half those of the first. Your actual contractions will feel the same, but the whole labor will be telescoped.

During the second, or *accelerated phase,* the waves of uterine contractions are higher, as you can see from the diagram, and the intervals between the contractions have shortened considerably. The length of one wave may be from 45 to 60 seconds by now, and the periods of rest are shorter, usually from 2 to 4 minutes.

The same study of the labor of many women has shown that the average length of time for the accelerated phase—the dilation of the cervix from about 3 to 8 centimeters or 1½ to 4 fingers—is about 3 to 4 hours.

The *transition* is the third phase of the first stage of labor. The contractions, represented as waves in our diagram, have become long, strong and erratic. They may have several peaks. They build up to maximum strength very quickly. They may last up to 1½ minutes, and the intervals between contractions are now shorter than the contractions themselves. The interval of rest may only be from 30 seconds to about 90 seconds. In fact, you may have just congratulated yourself that you managed to get through one of these contractions when you feel the next one already beginning. This, as you can imagine, is the hardest part of your labor. The only saving grace is that this phase is the shortest of the three subdivisions of the first stage of labor, and will usually last only from half an hour to an hour. I don't want to minimize the severity of the transitional contractions. You should be prepared for them and you should realize that this is like the final sprint of the uterine muscles. This period will demand more concentrated effort than any part previously experienced. But I will give you tools to work with and teach you how best to cope with this difficult part of your labor. One of my students reported to me one day on her labor. She said, "You talked of waves in labor, but it was a hurricane that hit me in transition."

The reason that I have given you approximate time limits for these phases of labor is to let you have some idea of what to expect. I cannot emphasize enough, however, that these are averages. There are many variations, all within the norm, and I want you to realize that it is very unlikely that your labor will be like any textbook description. Do not let this disturb you. In fact, it is one of the great advantages of the Lamaze technique that it provides the techniques to use as your individual labor demands. No two labors are the same. Even your own subsequent labors will differ and change in character from delivery to delivery.

THE FIRST TECHNIQUE OF BREATHING FOR THE FIRST STAGE OF LABOR

I will now give you three different breathing techniques to use during your first stage of labor. As you pass from preliminary labor, through accelerated labor, to the transition, you will adjust your breathing to the changes of the uterine contractions. I always think of this as if I were driving a car, shifting from first to second to third gear. It would never occur to you to

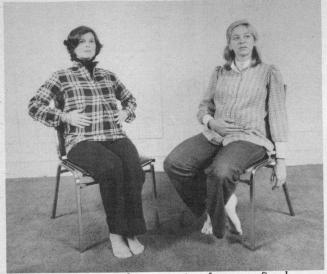

*To begin breathing practice, focus on fixed
object, breathe in through nose, out
through mouth; massage abdomen*

stay in first gear when you want to go faster. In the
same way, you will have to "shift gear" as your labor
progresses, in order to stay in control of your uterine
contractions.

And now to the first breathing technique you will
use in early labor. Be sure not to use this technique as
long as you can walk, talk or laugh through a contraction. You may get so excited at the onset of your
labor that you will want to breathe with it even if
there is no actual need. Please don't, because you will
soon become very bored by the whole process. Remember that the first phase can take hours and hours. You'd
be better off going for a walk with your husband, see-
ing a movie or tending to your usual house activities.
We often get so excited at the onset of labor that we

want to rush off to the hospital, hoping the baby will come quicker once we are there. Time, on the contrary, will seem endless if you arrive at the hospital too early. There is little in the labor room to divert your attention, and you may find this very demoralizing. At home, you will be more relaxed and fortified with the confidence your training has given you to handle the long latent part of labor. Of course, your own physician will give you exact instructions as to when he wants to be called. But my general advice is, don't rush.

Our aim during labor is to create a strong center of concentration through disciplined activity. The breathing technique we use has to be deliberate and different from our normal automatic breathing. I want you to breathe with your chest. Try it first by placing your hands flat under your breasts and letting your middle fingers meet. When you breathe with your chest, you will notice that your middle fingers will part slightly when you inhale and come together again when you exhale. Keep your abdomen relaxed while you breathe in this fashion. To make this chest breathing even more deliberate, I want you to inhale through your nose and exhale through your mouth. It's almost like whistling the air out. Take from 6 to 9 breaths in a minute, and count your breaths as you practice.

Begin every contraction by taking a deep cleansing breath. This will give you a good exchange of oxygen and carbon dioxide at the onset of a contraction, and at the same time relax you. Relaxation is a most important factor, as our usual reaction to a uterine contraction is what is called a "flight reaction." We tense our whole body. By taking a cleansing breath at the beginning of each contraction, you begin the contraction in a relaxed condition.

Now inhale through your nose, exhale through your lips, making a little noise with your breathing in order to keep a good rhythm. Count your breaths, and end each contraction with another cleansing breath. The relaxing breath at the end of each contraction is also of great importance. It means that you really come to a full stop, at the end of each contraction, emotionally and physically.

WHAT TO DO WITH YOUR HANDS

It's very difficult to know what to do with one's hands in labor. You certainly should not grip the sides of your bed or dig your fingernails into your husband's arm. In order to avoid such tension, do what comes naturally and soothe the pain by massaging your abdomen gently in time to your breathing. This is the best way to do it: Cupping your hands lightly, place them under your abdomen. Then massage gently with your fingertips, leading your arms out and up while you inhale, completing the circle down again as you exhale. This massage, or "effleurage" as it is called professionally, not only provides another point of concentration, but also feels good. A light massage will help to relieve the tension in your abdomen during a contraction. It actually has the same effect as rubbing a place on your body that hurts. You can also try to massage your abdomen with one hand, using your whole hand gently. Or you may like to let your partner gently massage your belly. He can sit at your side and, using the palm of his hand, massage your abdomen slowly.

If you have to use a fetal monitor, which requires two belts around your belly, one for monitoring the fetal heart, the other for monitoring the uterine contraction, it will be difficult to use your hands in a circular movement over your abdomen. However, you will find that a gentle massage just over the lowest part of your abdomen will feel very soothing.

HYPERVENTILATION

Occasionally you may feel a little dizzy when you practice this deliberate breathing technique. We call this hyperventilation, or what happens when the balance between the oxygen intake and the carbon dioxide output is disturbed. During a prolonged practice session you may even feel a tingling or stiffening in your hands and feet or around your lips. It is unlikely, however, that this will happen in labor, as your uterus will need a great deal of oxygen while it is contracting. But just in case, here are two easy ways to overcome this: Cup your hands, hold them over your nose and mouth and breathe in your own carbon dioxide; or hold your breath for a few seconds when the contraction is over. This will soon accumulate enough carbon dioxide, and your dizziness will quickly disappear. Hyperventilation is most likely to occur in labor during the *accelerated* and *transition* stages.

I suggest that if you become hyperventilated at the hospital and do not want to hold your breath, use a little paper sandwich bag to breathe into. This will be more effective than using your hands. And since you are going to bring this little paper bag along, there are a few things you can add to it which may be useful during labor. One of these is a small can of talcum powder. In actual labor you will be massaging your skin during each contraction. Your fingers may get hot and sticky. You may irritate your abdomen after a long period of massaging. Use the talcum powder on your abdomen or your hands to avoid such excessive friction. Let your partner sprinkle it on whenever you need it. (Later we'll discover many other things to carry along in our Lamaze bag.)

Keep your eyes open during a contraction and while practicing the breathing technique. Be sure, however, to focus on one point in the room. This will help you to concentrate. You will find that nothing happening outside your line of vision will concern you. It is vitally important to maintain this discipline in your practice session since during real labor you will need every ounce of concentration. An even better way would be to have eye contact with your partner. He could then work easily with you and correct your breathing when necessary. You may find that in practicing the eye contact with him, you'll probably break up laughing. But to tell the truth, I've never seen anybody laugh or giggle through labor, though I must admit that would be a great way to have a baby!

POSITION OF BODY DURING EARLY LABOR

You do not have to lie down when you are in labor. We always assume that the moment we go into the hospital we have to lie down in a bed and behave like a very sick person. I want you to remember that having a baby is a healthy event, and that the only reason we go to a hospital is because it is safer, not because we are suffering from a disease. I realize it isn't easy to overcome the notion that hospitals are places where one must suffer.

It is interesting to remember that forty to fifty years ago, when most women delivered their babies at home, nobody would have thought to call a laboring woman "a patient." She was just "a woman in labor" or "a woman giving birth to her child." It was only when women were encouraged to have their babies in hospitals that the laboring woman was called a "patient," a term that obviously makes us think of illness and suffering.

In fact, with the introduction of the episiotomy (a small surgical incision in the area between vagina and anus to allow the baby to emerge more easily and without tearing), having a baby actually became a surgical procedure.

Many hospitals insist that when you enter—having walked comfortably from your car or taxi into the hospital lobby—you must immediately get into a wheelchair. This may make you feel apprehensive straight away. You are likely to remember all the old tales of suffering in childbirth. But try to realize that once you enter the hospital, the hospital is responsible for your well-being. Even if you have to sit in a wheelchair, take the ride to the labor room in good humor and don't let it depress you.

In the labor room you will be asked to undress and put on a hospital gown, which is usually not attractive at all. I know you would much rather wear your own pretty gown. But remember that this hospital gown is functional, serves a good purpose and is far more practical to wear during labor than your own.

When the attending nurse asks you to get into bed, you will see a bed similar to yours at home (with just one pillow) although it may be a bit higher, for the convenience of the doctors and nurses. Don't forget that all hospital beds can be rolled up. Ask your nurse to roll it to any angle that is comfortable. Most of us can breathe much better with our heads raised, or even sitting up, and there is no reason you should not experiment in order to find your own comfortable position. You may want to lie on your side, sit up tailor fashion, legs crossed, or recline at any angle that suits you. You will only have to lie flat when you are being examined or when your physician suggests a certain position that he prefers you to be in.

MAN'S ROLE DURING PRACTICE

When you practice the first breathing technique at home, let your partner give you precise commands. He should have a stop watch with a sweep second hand to time you. Practice the breathing for approximately one minute—occasionally varying the time from 40 to 60 seconds to imitate the length of a real contraction. It is extremely important that your partner be as precise in his commands as you will have to be in your performance. Therefore he has to give the command: *contraction begins* and then *contraction ends,* and not just say "start" and "stop." This is important because you are training yourself to react to a uterine contraction with a respiratory response instead of a flight response. We are using therefore what is called "secondary conditioning," which means the correct command has to trigger your reaction.

It will also be helpful if your partner calls off the seconds while you practice your breathing. He should say: "Contraction begins," and then call out, "15 seconds . . . 30 seconds . . . 45 seconds . . . contraction ends." You will find this a very helpful device. It will make the contraction seem shorter. When your partner calls out 30 seconds, you will know that you are at the halfway point and when he says 45 seconds, it will mean "going, going, going, gone." Many couples find this not only useful during practice sessions, but also in actual labor. Your partner's signal at that time will be your cleansing breath. From this he will know that you have started another contraction. He will then look at his watch and call out the seconds for you. Try it and see how you like it.

Now let's practice the first breathing technique.

Take up any position that is comfortable for you. Contraction begins. Take a deep, relaxing, cleansing breath. Breathe in through your nose, and slowly exhale through your lips. Count your breaths, focus your eyes on a point in the room, or even better have eye contact with your partner, and massage your abdomen lightly with your fingertips, out and up as you inhale, down as you exhale. Or let your partner gently massage your abdomen. Finish with a deep cleansing breath.

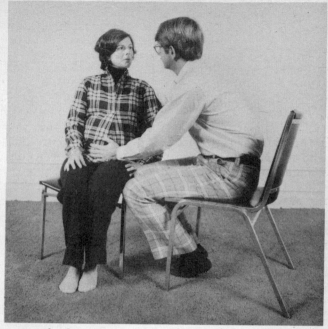

*It is both important and helpful for the partner to
supervise his partner while she practices her breathing*

Be sure to keep the rest of your body as relaxed as
possible while practicing.

When you practice by yourself, give yourself commands—contraction begins, contraction ends—and follow the time on a clock with a second hand. Also
visualize the pictures and diagrams that show contractions, so that it will be clear in your mind how your
body is working at the time. It always helps to imagine
the wave of a contraction and how you will ride the
wave with your breathing technique. And be sure to
practice your breathing with any Braxton-Hicks contraction that you may feel.

LESSON 4

What to do for back labor; breathing
techniques two and three, for the
accelerated and transitional phases; how
the partner can simulate a contraction

We will begin by reviewing what you have learned in the previous lessons. I expect you to carry on with the neuromuscular control exercises, so you can improve your body control and you and your partner can develop good teamwork. I am sure you will have noticed by now that the body-building exercises are no longer so tiring. In fact, you probably feel better for performing them and strengthening these muscles that have to carry most of the strain during pregnancy.

And now again to our first breathing technique. Do you think that by now you can describe our first technique to a friend who has never heard of it? You would have to begin by telling her that we divide the first stage of labor into three parts. They are: 1) The preliminary or latent part of labor, in which the cervix effaces and starts to dilate. 2) The accelerated part of labor, in which the cervix dilates approximately from 3 to 8 centimeters, or 1½ to 4 fingers. And, finally 3) The transition, in which the cervix dilates from approximately 8 to 10 centimeters, or 4 to 5 fingers. The waves of uterine contractions change in character as labor progresses, and you will remember that you must synchronize your breathing techniques with the intensity of the sensations that you will feel.

Then you must tell your friend what the actual breathing technique is like. We begin the contraction by taking a deep, relaxing, cleansing breath. This is followed by deliberate chest breathing, inhaling through the nose, exhaling through the mouth. We finish, when the contraction subsides, with another deep, relaxing, cleansing breath. We take any position that is comfortable, concentrating on one point in the room or having eye contact. At the same time we effleurage, or massage, our abdomen, moving our fingertips lightly in a circular motion to the rhythm of our breathing, or we encourage our partner to massage our abdomen gently.

Now try the breathing once again while I give the commands: Contraction begins. Take a deep, cleansing breath. Now breathe comfortably and deliberately with your chest, inhale through your nose, exhale through your mouth, 15 seconds, 30 seconds, 45 seconds . . . the contraction is over. End with a deep cleansing breath. Did you have between 6 and 9 breaths during this simulated contraction?

WHERE DO YOU FEEL A CONTRACTION?

I wonder if you have ever thought about where in your abdomen you will actually feel a contraction? Will you feel it all over, just low down, or perhaps in the back? Actually, the majority of women feel their labor low down, just above the pubic bone, but deep inside and spreading towards the groin. Some may feel a contraction beginning in the lower back and radiating to the lower abdomen, even drawing into the thighs. If you feel your labor in your legs, massage your legs! Don't get stuck rubbing your belly when most of the pain is in your thighs. Remember, I give you the tools to work with, but it will be up to you, according to your labor, to decide how and when you use the tools. All this demands a great flexibility on your part, but it also makes sense that you react to your body and its own rhythm instead of to what I have said or what you may have read in a textbook.

I remember being woken one morning by a telephone call. An excited voice was saying, "Mrs. Bing, Mrs. Bing, we are in the hospital and it's all in Charlotte's legs! What can we do?" I managed to open my eyes and say sleepily, "Massage her thighs." "Oh," said the voice on the other end of the line. Then I heard a click and I could see in my mind how he was racing upstairs to massage Charlotte's thighs. About twenty-five per cent of women experience what is called "back labor." I want you all to be aware of the fact that back labor exists. I am sure this may come as a surprise for many of you. After all, why should one feel anything in the back, when one imagines that the uterus is right here in front in the abdomen? Obviously the baby is there in front too, and the most natural thing would be to expect labor where one imagines the baby and uterus to be.

There is no one cause for back labor. However, it most often occurs when the baby lies in a posterior position: the baby is facing the mother's abdomen with the back of his head pressed against her spine. It is important, therefore, for you to be prepared for a possible experience of back labor.

WAYS TO ALLEVIATE BACK LABOR

Now what can we do about back labor? Your breathing technique should remain the same, whether you feel contractions in your abdomen or in your back. However, it is possible to alleviate the discomfort of back labor in a number of ways:

1. counter pressure
2. change of position
3. change of temperature

1. Instead of massaging your abdomen, you can massage or put pressure on your back. Back labor is usually felt in two distinct points low on your back, near the sacrum.

Massaging your back is fine, but does not really help you to relax. Your partner's help at this point will be invaluable. He can massage your back, or put counter pressure against the points that hurt during a contraction. He can put a good deal of pressure on your back and need not worry about hurting you at all. The uterus is far away from the area he will be pressing against. In fact, the more pressure he exerts against the painful areas, the better you will feel.

When your partner has been pressing his fists into your back for two hours or more, not only will his back be sore, but his knuckles will be rubbed through. We therefore suggest that you bring two tennis balls or a can of tennis balls to lean against and give your husband a rest. Actually, anything hard will do the trick. The tennis balls will give the counter pressure in your back and relieve some of the back pain.

Tell your partner he does not have to worry about finding the right spot to press against. You are sure to tell him in no uncertain terms to move his hand or fist to the left, to the right, to the middle, or up or down.

2. Change your position. What would you think the aim in changing position to be? The simple answer is: Get the baby off your back! As long as you are half sitting or perhaps even lying on your back, you have the weight of the baby on your spine, which definitely aggravates back labor. You will probably find it far more comfortable to lie on your side, allowing the weight of the baby to be carried by the bed. Bend both knees, placing the upper knee in front of the lower one, and support the upper knee with a pillow. It is best to lie on the side of the "occiput," which means the side where the back of the baby's head is. If you cannot tell where the baby's head is, do not hesitate to ask the attending nurse or your physician. You may also feel perfectly comfortable sitting up at an angle of 90 degrees. Have your husband roll up your bed, but do not lean against the back of the bed. Round your back and put a pillow for support against the lower part of your spine.

Another position which some women find helpful is what we call the "knee-chest" position. You kneel and rest your body on your lower arms and hands. In this position the weight of the baby is entirely off your spine, and may provide excellent relief from all back pressure. Many women also use this position when suffering from severe menstrual cramps. A very good variation here would be to kneel on the bed and at the same time to lean against the rolled-up bed. In this position, the weight of the baby would be off your spine, gravity would help to move the baby down, and the pressure of the baby's head against the cervix might help the dilation. Try out these positions and practice the breathing exercises with them—this way you will be prepared for any changes that may occur during your labor.

You could also sit on the edge of the bed, feet resting on a chair. Use the bed table with a pillow to rest your arms and shoulders. This will be less tiring than the kneeling position.

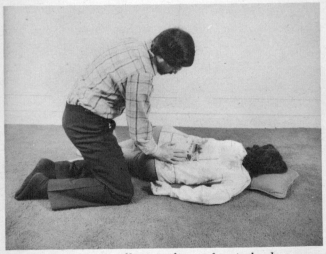

One way to alleviate discomfort in back
labor is to lie on your side with partner
exerting pressure on lower back

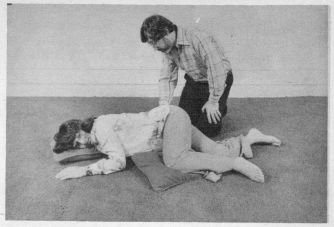

When taking the side position for back
labor, be sure to bend both knees
and elevate the upper leg to avoid stress

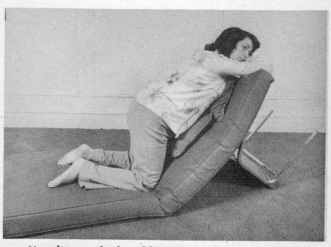

Kneeling on bed and leaning against raised head
of bed is an excellent position for back labor

3. While you are still at home, during the early stages of labor, you may find a heating pad or hot-water bottle very beneficial for back labor. I am afraid we are usually not allowed to use heating pads in the hospital.

In the hospital you could use a coolpack or Scotch ice or any of the picnic coolers that you can freeze beforehand in the freezing compartment of your refrigerator. Freezing, i.e., anesthetizing the area that hurts with a cold compress, may relieve back pain.

All these methods alleviate the discomfort of back labor. You will have to experiment once you are in labor and discover which method is best for you.

SECOND BREATHING TECHNIQUE

We will now discuss the second part of the first stage of labor, a period during which the cervix dilates from 3 to 8 centimeters. Contractions are now becoming stronger, they last from 45 to 60 seconds, the intervals are now less than 5 minutes, most likely between 2 and 3 minutes. First-phase breathing is usually no longer effective once contractions have reached this accelerated pace. You will now need a second tool to control the strong waves. Let's say we have to shift into second gear.

Our aim must be to speed up the breathing, making it much more shallow, as if beginning a fast sprint. If one starts running, one's breathing speeds up. In this accelerated phase, the uterus works harder, and you must react to this with more rapid breathing. This allows the hard-working uterine muscle to function more efficiently and also to bring more oxygen to the uterus and to your baby.

I want to give you a few pointers before you try out this faster, shallow breathing.

Start, as always, with a deep, relaxing, cleansing breath. You can do this breathing either through your mouth or through your nose. The advantage of practicing it through your nose is that your throat and mouth will not get so dry. It is up to you however. If you try breathing through your mouth, keep both passages open so that you will always feel a little air coming through your nose as well. This helps a great deal in relaxing the facial muscles. Breathe lightly and evenly, accentuating your exhalation slightly. You will find that the inhalation is a reflex; but you will have to concentrate on making the exhalation short and staccato, so that your breaths stay shallow and even. Breathe quietly; in fact, don't make any noise at all.

Remember to keep your neck muscles relaxed. Open your mouth very slightly, almost as if you were smiling. This will help you do this breathing almost in your throat.

Try this breathing technique very slowly at first. It may help you to beat a rhythm with your fingers. It has also helped some women to breathe in certain rhythms, stressing every first breath in four—for example, a little song in 4/4 rhythm. I've found that "Yankee Doodle" gives a wonderful beat to breathe too. Be sure to make the "Yankee Doodle" very "moderato." If you find yourself going "allegro vivace," you can be sure your breathing is much too fast. I'd rather have you err on the slow side than breathe too fast.

Don't be too ambitious when you first try this breathing technique. It is easy to become discouraged. Remember that it is quite difficult, and must be practiced over a long period of time. I would advise you to try it several times a day. Begin by doing it for 15 seconds only, then increase it to 30 seconds. Eventually you should be able to breathe easily and evenly for about 45 seconds to a minute without undue fatigue. If you lose the rhythm, overexpand your chest by breathing in more air than you breathe out, or if you get tired, blow out all the air in your lungs and resume the breathing immediately. Always begin and end your practice with a cleansing breath.

SECOND BREATHING
TECHNIQUE IN LABOR

Now I am going to show you how to apply this new breathing technique in labor.

Look again at the diagram showing the second part of the first stage of labor, the accelerated phase. The waves representing intensity of contraction are fairly high. You will see from the drawing that each wave increases in intensity as it rises and decreases in intensity as it subsides.

Your task at this point is to follow the wave of the contraction. There is no sense in exhausting yourself by breathing rapidly from beginning to end of the wave. Remember that one of our main objectives is to channel our energies and be as economical as possible with our muscle power.

You must therefore start the contraction with a cleansing breath and then start to breathe slowly, increasing your rate of breathing as the contraction increases in intensity. Breathe in a 4/4 rhythm at the peak of the contraction, but immediately slow down your breathing as the contraction tapers off. Conclude with another cleansing breath. In this way you will stay with the wave, accelerating when the contraction builds up and decelerating as it subsides. It is as if you are running a race with the contraction, but a race in which you must only keep parallel.

I will now give you the commands for this second breathing technique. Contraction begins: focus your eyes on one point or have eye contact with your partner. Take a cleansing breath and relax your whole body. Start to breathe slowly but take shallow breaths. Now the contraction is getting stronger, stronger, stronger. It is at its peak. It is still at its peak. It is still there. It is still there, and now it begins to subside, slower and slower and slower and slower. Contraction is over. Take a deep cleansing breath.

After you have practiced accelerating and decelerating your breathing for a few days, I want you to add the effleurage, or massage of your abdomen. This is difficult and needs a great deal of coordination, as the massage has to be performed slowly, regularly and lightly, as your breathing builds up and slows down.

When practicing this breathing by yourself, I want you to give exact commands in your own mind. Watch a clock with a second hand, and say to yourself "Contraction begins!" Then slowly increase your rate of breathing so that you get to the peak within 10 to 15 seconds, stay at the peak for about 20 to 30 seconds, slow down for 15 to 20 seconds. Conclude by saying "Contraction ends!"

YOUR PARTNER SIMULATES A CONTRACTION

If your partner practices with you, let him put his hand just above your knee, and as he gives you the command "Contraction begins!" let him put pressure on your thigh. He should increase the pressure slowly, coming to the peak of his pressure in about 10 to 15 seconds, keeping it up for about 20 to 30 seconds, then reducing the pressure slowly for about another 15 to 20 seconds.

In this way we are simulating, in a sense, a uterine contraction. You will be reacting to an actual physical discomfort which increases in intensity, comes to a peak and decreases again. Try it. After you have tried this, ask your partner to press your leg once while you're not panting, just as hard as he did it before. I am sure you will discover that the pressure is quite a painful sensation without your breathing technique.

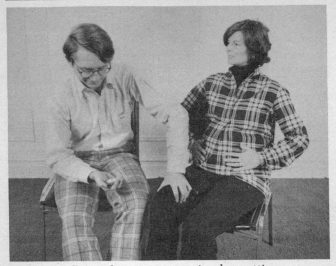

*Bill simulates a contraction by putting
hard pressure above Gail's knee.
Correct breathing eliminates her discomfort*

Practice in different positions in order to be prepared for labor and be sure to be absolutely relaxed at all times. Also remind your partner to watch you closely, and correct any mistakes he sees.

THE TRANSITION

You will remember that during the transition period the cervix dilates from about 7 or 8 centimeters to 10 centimeters, or 3½ or 4 to 5 fingers. The contractions are now more severe than at any previous time. Before I tell you about the breathing for the transition period, I want to mention some symptoms that may occur during this phase of your labor.

1. Frequently there is a bloody, mucous discharge at

this time. Nurses often call this a "good bloody show." This is caused by pressure from the baby's head against the cervix, which is extremely sensitive and has many delicate, superficial blood vessels. These little blood vessels may break. You will suddenly notice that you are getting rather wet. It is important for you and your partner to know that a "bloody show" at this point is normal. In fact it is a sign that the baby's head is descending and that you are getting closer to full dilation, and the second stage of labor.

2. Most women will feel an increasing amount of pressure in the rectum at this point. You may also have back labor, even if up to now you have felt labor only in your lower abdomen. You may find that sitting upright and leaning slightly forward will alleviate a great deal of back pressure, or perhaps even lying on your side. Also, instead of massaging your abdomen, put your hands over your coccyx (the lowest vertebra of your spine) and press hard. Better still, let your partner press upward against your coccyx.

3. It is possible that you will already feel a slight desire to push at this point. However, it is most important that you do not push until your physician has examined you and given explicit permission to do so. The desire to push is a reflex set off by pressure of the baby's head against the vaginal walls, the rectum and the pelvic floor. Occasionally this reflex occurs before you are fully dilated. It is imperative, therefore, that you act against this reflex and don't push until dilation is complete. If you try to push the baby through an opening that is too small, you will have unnecessary pain, you will waste a great deal of valuable effort and you will risk a swelling of your cervix.

There is a very easy way to counteract the urge to push. It can be done by forcibly exhaling, or blowing out air until the urge has passed. You know, of course, that when you try to expel a stool, you hold your breath. Even if you are lifting a heavy weight, you hold your breath to do so.

Try the following exercise: Hold your breath and strain. Now blow out continuously, always breathing in *and* out, and try to strain at the same time. Notice that this is almost impossible. You will understand now why I ask you to blow out forcibly and continually during labor whenever you get an early urge to push and have been told not to.

4. Some women feel nauseated during transition and may even vomit. Please realize that if this should happen to you, these unpleasant symptoms are within the normal course of events. Don't be frightened if they occur.

5. Occasionally a woman will start to shake or tremble. You may find that it becomes more and more difficult to relax. You may feel hot and cold, and your control of the uterine waves may become more and more difficult.

I would like to tell you about one of my students whom I had warned about these possible unpleasant symptoms during the transition period. Apparently she had not really believed that anything like that could happen to her. But there she was in transition, her legs shaking like a leaf. She didn't become frightened, but she thought it was so funny that she started to laugh. She kept on pointing at her trembling legs and laughing. The nurse in attendance thought my student had lost her mind. She had certainly never before seen anybody laugh during the transition.

6. Finally, there is one more symptom I want to mention. Almost every woman gets terribly irritable during this phase of labor. Up to now you have been grateful for your partner's help: his rubbing your back, wetting your lips with a sponge, encouraging you. Now suddenly you may find yourself snapping at him: "Don't touch me. Don't talk to me, leave me alone!" Partners must be aware of this possibility and remember that this bad temper is only temporary. It will disappear as soon as you are fully dilated and have been given permission to push.

BREATHING
DURING TRANSITION

In order to stay in control during these extremely strong contractions, we need a new breathing technique which is even more precise and demands even more concentrated effort on our part. A stronger, more forceful rhythm has to be established. As an obstetrician once observed, "You have to become Rockettes in labor," which means that you have to work with the kind of precision the Rockettes use in Radio City Music Hall. We can do this best by using four or six or eight short breaths, followed by a quick exhalation (through pursed lips), continuing this pattern until the end of the contraction, which may now last as long as 1½ minutes.

The short exhalation after 4, 6, or 8 breaths should be just like a short accent. Be sure to make it quite short—don't rest on it by breathing too slowly. Do not forget to use the cleansing breath here at the beginning and end of the contraction. These strong transition contractions are likely to reach the peak of their intensity within 1 or 2 seconds of the beginning, so you will have no time to accelerate slowly. Use the very rapid breathing immediately after the cleansing breath, and only slow down when the contraction begins to taper off. Do not massage your abdomen any more during this period, but do have a specific place for your hands. Support your abdomen with them, for example, putting slight pressure on your groin. Or you may prefer pressing your hands against your coccyx.

Should you feel a desire to push during such a contraction, blow out continuously, remembering to breathe in after each forcible exhalation. Then return to the breathe-and-blow pattern, once the urge to push has subsided, for as long as the contraction continues.

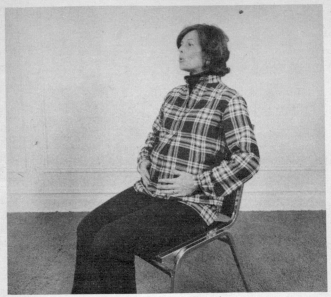

Gail practices third breathing technique
by establishing a strict pattern;
6 quick breaths followed by a short blow

I suggest that you use the transition breathing once your contractions begin to come as rapidly as 1½ minutes apart, regardless of whether you experience any of the other symptoms mentioned above.

Remember that you must react to your specific uterine contractions and not to a preconceived idea of what your labor should be like. Let me repeat again: every labor is different from every other. You may experience innumerable variations of my description of labor. But the great advantage of the Lamaze technique is that it provides you with enough techniques to stay in control of your labor, however it may vary from your expectations.

I will now give the command: Contraction begins; cleansing breath; rapid breathing—1, 2, 3, 4, 5, 6, exhale (*do not blow out too much air or you may hyperventilate*) 1, 2, 3, 4, 5, 6, blow out, 1, 2, 3, etc.

Contraction over, cleansing breath . . . and rest. Make the most of the rest between contractions. Save energy!

Here is some advice to the coach. It happens frequently that your partner will suddenly say, "I've had enough, I'm giving up, I can't make it" or something to that effect. Go and get the nurse or doctor and ask him or her to examine your wife. The chances are she is either fully dilated or 5–10 minutes away from it.

The untrained woman will feel like giving up at 5 or 6-centimeter dilation. The trained woman will want to quit when she is almost ready to push her baby out.

This rapid breathing will make you thirsty, particularly if you breathe through your mouth. Many hospitals will not allow you to drink anything during labor except an occasional sip of water. If you are lucky you may be offered some crushed ice. I advise you, therefore, to bring some lollipops or a peppermint stick to the hospital, so that you can lubricate your mouth a little between contractions.

You can bring a "Lamaze bag," which can, of course, be any old shopping bag, and which will hold your can of talcum powder, the lollipops or peppermint sticks, a small paper bag to breathe in in case you hyperventilate, and some other items which you will find on the complete list on page 112.

LESSON 5

The second stage of labor; what happens during actual delivery and how to prepare for it; partner's role during delivery; how to stop pushing on command

We have now covered the entire first stage of labor, and you have learned the techniques that will be used during this long period. Before discussing the second stage, or *expulsion*, it is imperative to review all our exercises, relaxation techniques and breathing methods.

Do you remember what to do if you have back labor? You will recall that the breathing techniques remain the same whether your labor is felt in your abdomen or your back, and that there are changes of position that will help. You should roll your bed up to an angle of 90 degrees. Do not lean back, but bend slightly forward, and put a pillow against your lower back. This will help to take the weight of the baby off your spine. You may prefer instead to try lying on your side, your upper knee resting on a pillow over the lower knee. Another technique is the knee-chest position, in which you lean forward on all fours with your lower arms resting on a pillow, or one in which you kneel on the bed, leaning your arms and trunk against the raised bed. Or sit on the edge of your bed, feet resting on a chair, and support your arms and shoulders on a table.

We have also seen how you can ease back labor by exerting pressure on your lower back with your fingers or fists. Or your partner may massage you, pressing his hands as hard as he can against the lower part of your spine. Or you can use the tennis balls you brought along in your "Lamaze bag."

If you have back labor during transition, the kneeling position, leaning against the raised bed, may be most comfortable. But in the final analysis, it will always have to be you who decides which position, counter pressure or cold application is the most comforting at the time. If there is a great deal of rectal pressure, ask your partner or the nurse to push against your coccyx. Remember that about 25 per cent of women experience back labor, so it's important to be well prepared for this possibility.

Now practice the three breathing techniques for the first stage of labor. I'm sure you will notice how much you've improved in the week or two that you have been practicing. The rapid shallow breathing should be easier to perform, your rhythm should be better—and now you probably don't get too exhausted. During the stress of actual labor your breathing will come quite easily—automatically, in fact. All your practice and training will help you to coordinate your activities, channel your energy and use your body with a minimum amount of effort.

THE SECOND STAGE OF LABOR

Expulsion is really the most wonderful stage of labor. Until now you've worked hard, concentrating on riding each wave of your contractions. You've had to relax under great stress and still perform your breathing techniques. And all this has probably gone on for a good number of hours.

During the second stage you will *still* have to work tremendously hard. But now you can help your uterus in the expulsion of your baby. It is the most satisfying and exhilarating work you will ever have to do. This stage is much shorter than the long, tedious dilation of the cervix, and you know that your baby will soon be born. You will feel during this period as if you have a second wind. Although the expulsion will be just about the hardest physical work you'll ever do in your life, it will feel absolutely wonderful.

Before I explain the technique of pushing, I want you to look again at the illustration showing the expulsion of the baby, so that you will understand the workings of your uterus, how the baby is being rotated and how you can help with the expulsion—consciously, in order to expel your baby smoothly. You will be able to do this, because you have been practicing the pelvic floor exercises for many weeks.

At this point you will see again how important the Kegel exercises have been to prepare your body for the expulsion of your baby.

Once the baby is descending, there will be great pressure on your rectum. It is now imperative for you to be able to relax the pelvic floor.

WHAT HAPPENS
DURING DELIVERY

Look once again at the illustrations and visualize how the baby is expelled from the uterus. Think also of how you can help with your own pushing to bring the baby out as smoothly and quickly as possible. You can see that as the baby enters the vagina, or birth canal, it rotates 90 degrees, and now faces the mother's spine. The baby's head bends down when it reaches the pelvic floor, so that the crown of its head shows first at the exit of the vagina, or vulva. You can see now why the doctor will talk of "the baby's head crowning."

If it is your first baby you will start pushing in the labor room and be moved to the delivery room only when about a dime-sized area of the head is showing. At this point your husband will probably be able to tell you what color hair the baby has. To push the baby down this far may take anywhere from 10 to 30 minutes. Then—in the delivery room—the baby's head will bend back as it stretches the outlet of the vagina, and you will push it out. This should take another 15 to 20 minutes, assuming that there are no complications. If this is your second or third or even fourth pregnancy, you will be moved into the delivery room as soon as you are fully dilated and have been given permission to push.

Now you'll need the action of the diaphragm to give additional force to the uterus in its expulsive action. You can reinforce the uterus by using your upper abdominal muscles, and by forcing down the diaphragm to help from above. Pushing the baby out is like piston action: hard pressure from above pushing down and out. Your aim now is to reduce the intra-abdominal space and to increase the intra-abdominal pressure.

This action could be best accomplished if you were allowed to assume a squatting position to expel the baby. It is interesting that about two-thirds of the women on our earth *still* give birth in the squatting position. I think we would never have to teach a woman to bear down if we could let her push the baby out while squatting. Unfortunately, modern society and modern obstetric technique demand of us that we push lying down, really against gravity and against normal instinct. Of course, it is easier for the attending physician to deal with any difficulties that may occur if the woman is lying on her back with legs raised. However, position and even designs for delivery tables are now slowly changing; that is to say, changing in such a way that the comfort of the delivering mother is considered. A new concept, the Lamaze labor-delivery-bed, has been accepted by now in a number of hospitals all over the country.

Such a labor-delivery-bed would not only allow the mother to labor and deliver in one bed and one place, which would afford her a far more effective and smoother effort, especially during the delivery of her baby, but it would also allow her to have her back raised and supported and to have her legs supported at a level lower than is possible on a regular delivery table. Her position would be something like this.

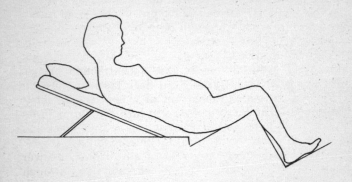

You can see how much more logical and physiologically sound such a position would be, and also how much more comfortable the mother would be. Surely, no other mammal on this earth is asked to give birth lying flat on its back with its legs up in the air!

But as the majority of women will still have to start their pushing in the labor room and then be moved onto a regular delivery table once a little of the head is showing, I will explain to you now how to practice the pushing in the labor bed.

Practice Pushing at Home for the Labor Room

Lean against your partner's legs, sitting on your tail bone at an angle of about 75 degrees from the horizontal. Rest your feet on the floor, feet and knees comfortably separated. Hold on to your knees or under your knees. Keep your elbows well out and push your head forward. Your back should be rounded as it is resting against your partner's legs.

It is important that you push correctly and in a disciplined fashion so that you can expel the baby in as short a period as possible. You will have to push only with contractions and only when you have been given the okay for pushing by some one in authority, i.e., a nurse, a resident or your doctor.

The contractions will slow down somewhat when you start to push. They will probably not be as violent as your transition contraction. Don't rush into pushing. You will be more effective if you do it slowly and deliberately. Now, let us assume a contraction begins. As usual, we start by taking a deep cleansing breath. However, to get the most out of a contraction, let it build up strength first before you help the uterus in its expulsion effort. Therefore, take a second cleansing breath. Then inhale a third time deeply, let out a little of your breath, hold the remaining air, relax your lower jaw and push steadily, directing all your force through your vagina. Remember, elbows out, head forward, pelvic floor muscles relaxed. Sustain the pushing effort for 10–15 seconds, let the air out, lower your head, quickly take another breath, exhale a little, hold the rest and bear down, relax your lower jaw, hold and push for 10–15 seconds, breathe out and let your head relax. Quickly take a third breath, exhale a little, hold the rest, relax your lower jaw, and push smoothly for 10–15 seconds, thinking in the direction of your vagina. Finally breathe out, and take several cleansing breaths to make up for the oxygen you didn't bring to the baby while you were pushing.

In this way you are helping the uterus by giving it direction and added force from above, while at the same time removing resistance from below. This is extremely hard work!

You can practice the pushing exercise safely every day, holding your breath for 10–15 seconds only. During actual labor, however, you will have to sustain your pushing efforts for a longer period. Usually you'll need three breaths and three pushes for one contraction. And in actual labor you will reinforce your uterus with deliberate muscular efforts. Each time you push, the baby will descend a certain distance, and each time the contraction is over the baby will slip back a little. It's really like taking two steps forward and one back. Therefore, the more force you can exert against the uterus from above and the more you can relax your pelvic-floor muscles from below, the faster your baby will be born.

PARTNER'S ROLE DURING EXPULSION

Your partner can be of great assistance in practicing this technique. He can make sure you are in a correct position. He can support your back. He can practice with you and give the pushing commands: "Breathe in —breathe out, breathe in—breathe out, breathe in—let out a litle air—hold your remaining breath, hold on to your legs, open them wide, keep your elbows out, raise your head, relax your lower lip, and push, push, push . . . breathe out—take a second breath, let out a little, hold your breath, relax your lower jaw and push . . . push . . . breathe out, quickly once more: breathe in, let out a little—hold, relax your lower lip and push, push . . . breath out and relax."

I have found that even the best-trained woman may forget how to push. The doctor gives her the permission to push with the next contraction, and she will suddenly look up in utter panic and say: "I've forgotten how!" It is unlikely that both of you will forget the same things at the same time, and it will help you enormously if your partner can give you exact commands. You'll have to tell him when the contraction begins, and he will then give you the signals when to breathe and push. I am sure that once he has done this for two or three contractions, you'll be able to function perfectly well on your own.

Try not to be too much of a perfectionist in labor. It may take you a few contractions until you really feel that you are pushing well. Don't be discouraged. You will fall into the correct pattern of pushing very quickly, particularly if you and your partner have trained together and are allowed to work together during labor and delivery.

THE DELIVERY-ROOM TABLE

The pushing technique that you will use on the delivery table is the same that you used in the labor room. The delivery-room table is very much like the table in your doctor's office: hard, flat and narow. But instead of putting your heels into stirrups, as you do in your doctor's office, your legs will be supported under your knees and thighs. This is much more comfortable. Unfortunately, in most hospitals the delivery table cannot be raised so that you can push down from above. You should therefore ask your doctor if you may bring your pillows from the labor room into the delivery room to support your shoulders and head. A few hospitals may provide a backrest on the delivery table or a foam-rubber bolster.

You will have handles or grips to hold onto, or you may hold the vertical bars that attach the stirrups to the table. These handles or bars will enable you to pull yourself up when you have to push.

In order to allow for the most comfortable position to push, ask that the stirrups be lowered, so that you can raise your back to an angle of about 40–45 degrees. If the table cannot be raised, or if there is no backrest available, push the pillows you've brought from the labor room well under your back, not just under your head and shoulders.

It is of great advantage to practice pushing in the actual positions you're likely to use during real labor. In this way, you can train your body and muscles to function well in the proper positions from the very beginning.

When you are on the delivery table your legs and your abdomen will be draped with sterile material. Be sure never to touch the sterile drapes! Keep your hands firmly on the bars. It used to be common to strap a woman's wrists in order to make sure that she would not inadvertently touch the sterile drapes placed over her abdomen and legs. However, most physicians and nurses will not insist on restraining your hands. They know that a trained woman will not touch any drapes or sheets she has been asked not to touch. It will be difficult for you to watch the emergence of your child, because you are too low and the drape obstructs your view. But frequently there is a mirror above the delivery table, which can be easily adjusted so that you can watch your baby being born.

HOW TO STOP PUSHING ON COMMAND

At the moment your baby's head emerges and begins rotating to allow the shoulders to come out, your doctor may tell you to stop pushing. It is of the utmost importance that you are prepared to cooperate immediately. Lean back, relax your body and blow out repeatedly until the urge to push is over. In a short time your doctor will advise you to continue pushing for the shoulders, but this pause is likely to be a difficult moment for you. The urge to push will probably be extremely strong and you will be asked to counteract this strong involuntary feeling. It's quite possible to prepare for this moment if, in your expulsion exercises at home, you let your husband occasionally give you the command "stop pushing," and you learn to react instantaneously.

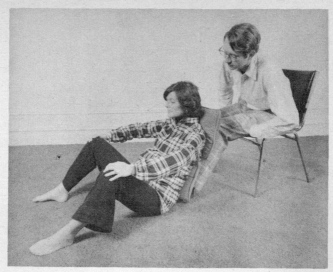

*Gail and Bill practice the labor room pushing
with Gail's back at about a 75° angle*

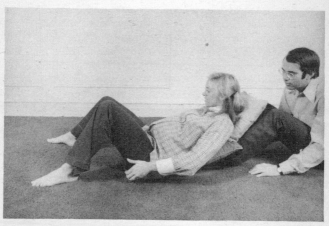

*Barbara and Tom practice the delivery room pushing
with Barbara's back at about a 35° angle*

LESSON 6

Recognizing real labor; what to bring
along; moment-to-moment at the hospital;
breathing with your labor; use of
medication; the great moment and after

I'm sure you have often wondered: How will I know when my labor begins? How will I be able to tell the difference between the kind of contractions I've been having for the last few weeks and the real ones? I've heard that perhaps I can sleep through part of my labor —is this true?

These are very legitimate questions. One good basic rule to follow is this: when you feel slight contractions and you are not sure whether this is real labor or not, the chances are it is *not*. Yes, you can sleep through early labor, but any contraction that doesn't wake you is obviously so mild that you don't have to concentrate on it. I have often found that the doctor and the laboring mother do not agree on when labor started. For the woman, it feels like labor when the contractions are obvious enough for her to be aware of them. They may be mild, but she is excited, she knows she should not eat any more, and she listens carefully to every little sign and symptom her body gives her. Finally she wants to know for certain and calls the doctor, who may tell her to come to the hospital to be examined. She arrives at the hospital and is examined, and the doctor tells her that she is not in labor yet.

This is very upsetting. She has been having contractions for hours by now, she has not eaten anything, she has been awake most of the night, and now the doctor tells her that this is not labor yet. What are those contractions, and when will they become effective so that the cervix begins to dilate? she asks herself. She is already tired, and the doctor tells her she has not even started labor yet. This can be a difficult time.

There are, however, certain definite indications that you should be aware of. Therefore I would like to discuss with you now the signs with which we associate the beginning of labor.

1. You may observe an increase in mucous discharge towards the end of your pregnancy. At one point this discharge will probably be tinged with a little blood. This will indicate the expulsion of the mucous plug which closes the cervix during your pregnancy. It is generally just a very slight stain, which you will notice only when you go to the bathroom. If no other symptoms—such as contractions or breaking of the membrane—occur simultaneously, don't get too excited at this point. It may be hours or even days before you will go into real labor. Therefore, losing the mucous plug is not necessarily a reliable indication of the beginning of labor.

2. The second indication of the beginning of labor is the onset of actual contractions. Contractions do not always start as the textbooks tell us: first about 20 minutes apart, gradually getting closer together and becoming more regular. It is just as normal for the contractions to begin only 5 minutes apart. Do not become alarmed if this occurs. It is a perfectly normal variation. It *is* important that you keep track of the intensity of the contractions, noting whether they last 30 seconds or more and if the intervals between them become shorter.

Although the uterine muscle is an involuntary muscle—like your heart or stomach—it is affected by your emotions. Just as you feel your heart beating violently if you are frightened or upset, or your stomach "turning over" if you are very nervous, so your uterus also reacts to anxieties. If you become very excited and tense, it may contract repeatedly—but, unfortunately, with no results. Therefore, your understanding of the process of labor will help you immensely in approaching your delivery. You can avoid unnecessary tension and allow your body to work smoothly during your labor. This understanding and knowledge will also help you give the doctor an accurate description of what's happening when you contact him at the onset of labor. (Your physician will always give you exact instructions as to when he wants to be called and when he wants you to leave for the hospital.)

BREAKING OF WATER

Breaking of water, or rupturing the membranes that contain the amniotic fluid in which the baby lives during your pregnancy, may occur at any time during your labor. You may become aware of a slow leaking or feel a sudden gush of fluid. This amniotic fluid is transparent and is therefore easily distinguishable from urine. You may have noticed, toward the end of your pregnancy, that you occasionally have difficulty in controlling your urine. A sudden sneeze, a laugh or cough can make it difficult for you to hold back the urine. But you *can* control it, whereas if your membranes leak, you cannot stop the escaping fluid by contracting your muscles. This will be a positive indication that the fluid you are losing is amniotic fluid and not urine. (Since your membranes may break while you are in bed, it's a good idea to put a rubber or plastic sheet on your mattress about a week before your due date.)

I'm sure your doctor will have given you instructions to call him as soon as your membranes break. He'll probably ask you to go to the hospital immediately, even if you have not yet felt any contractions. He wants you under hospital care so that no infection can occur once the membranes are ruptured.

Let me assure you that breaking of the membranes is entirely painless and that there is no definite time when you will lose this amniotic fluid. It's even possible that your physician will have to break the bag of waters artificially during your labor.

If your membranes break early in labor, it does not mean that you will have a "dry labor." Actually the fluid that you lose at the beginning of labor is only the tiny amount between the widest diameter of the baby's head and the cervix. Most of the fluid will be plugged off by the baby's head and shoulders. Don't worry if additional water escapes from time to time, especially during a contraction. The uterus keeps making more water, so there will be plenty left for the baby to remain cushioned and to help it finally emerge.

WHAT TO DO WHEN CONTRACTIONS BEGIN

If contractions start at night and are mild and far apart, try to rest as much as possible. Sleep between contractions as much as you can, so that you are well rested when your labor becomes more active and demands undivided attention. You can be sure that strong, advanced contractions will keep you awake, so make the most of your rest and ignore the beginning of labor as long as you can.

It may be impossible to sleep, however. That's very understandable, too. After all, you have been waiting anxiously for this moment for a long time. But I suggest that you do not lie awake in the dark. Get out of bed and take a comfortable bath in relaxing warm water. If the bath has been banned, take a shower. Then go to the kitchen and make yourself some tea and drink it with lots of sugar or honey. The tea is a stimulant and the sugar is energy-giving. If, after all this activity, you find that labor is progressing—the contractions are increasing in frequency and intensity—you will have to be up anyhow. If, on the other hand, your contractions have slowed down again and there seems to be little change in their character, go back to bed and sleep. You'll probably be very tired in the middle of the night, and sleep may come fairly easily once you have reassured yourself that you can be in control of the situation. Don't wake your husband until you need his help and support. He will better be able to do his part if he is well rested, too.

If labor starts during the day, cut down your intake of food and fluids.

May I suggest that you prepare some Jello a few days before your due date and keep it in the refrigerator. Jello is an ideal snack early in labor. Should you become hungry, broth and light food such as fruit or crackers will also help you if the beginning of labor is long. Do not drink any more milk. Remember that milk is a whole food and that it is hard to digest once labor has started.

Once labor has started in earnest your digestive system automatically stops working. Anything you eat remains undigested in the stomach. I am sure you have noticed even now, during your pregnancy, how distressed you can feel after a meal. There simply is not enough space any more. You can imagine how much more uncomfortable it will be if your stomach stops working. A full stomach may cause vomiting during labor. And should you for any reason require an inhalation anesthetic, it will be infinitely easier to have it on an empty stomach.

I'd like to suggest here that for about one to two weeks before your due date, you have your last meal of the day no later than 7:30 or 8:00 P.M.—and avoid midnight snacks.

Do not immediately lie down when labor begins. If you had a good night's rest go on with your regular activities without tiring yourself. Call your husband home, if he has already left for work. It will be much nicer for you to have him there than to wonder whether he can make it back in time to take you to the hospital.

Do not start any deliberate breathing during contractions until you absolutely feel the need for it. As long as you can walk or talk through a contraction, there is no need to use any specific breathing technique. You'll probably feel a strong temptation to start the deliberate breathing too early, out of pure enthusiasm and excitement that you are at long last in labor. But labor will seem endless if you start controlling it before there is any actual need. You'll tire yourself needlessly, wasting valuable energy that you'll need once labor progresses and the contractions demand concentrated control. Always remember that you must channel your energies, and that from the beginning to the end of your labor you will use the techniques that you have learned, deliberately and with considerable self-discipline.

WHAT TO TAKE
TO THE HOSPITAL

Pack your suitcase at least two weeks before due date. If you're going to nurse the baby, pack two nursing bras. Be sure that you do not buy nursing bras that come with a protective pad. These pads are usually made of some kind of plastic and do not allow for ventilation. The hospital will provide you with gauze pads for protection. (You can buy boxes of these pads at any drugstore, but you might find it cheaper to use old handkerchiefs or cut up an old sheet once you're home again.) Put two or three shorty nightgowns into your suitcase and, if you plan to nurse, be sure that the nightgowns open in front. This will enable you to nurse your baby without having to slip out of your nightgown at each feeding. Pack two belts for your sanitary napkins (the napkins themselves will be provided by the hospital) and a robe and slippers. Do not use tampons until you've had your post-partum examination and your doctor has given you permission. Have a separate bag ready for clothes and diapers for the baby. Put out the clothes you want to wear going home, so your husband won't have a last-minute search through closets and drawers. And don't expect to fit into your tightest skirts or dresses right away.

CONTENTS OF
THE LAMAZE BAG

Do you remember the Lamaze bag I told you to take to the hospital? Here is the list of things to put into your Lamaze bag:

1. A bottle of champagne or wine to celebrate with doctors and nurses after you've given birth. Also bring some plastic glasses, for there are never enough in the hospital. Ask the nurse to put the champagne on ice when you arrive at the hospital, so it will be nice and cool when you need it.

2. Some food for your partner or coach. This is especially useful if you happen to labor at night. Few hospitals have food at nightime, and your partner will get ravenously hungry, because he is working every moment of your labor with you. Luckily, you yourself will not be hungry during labor; also, you won't be allowed to eat. But once you've given birth, you will probably be very hungry. So tell your partner to save a sandwich for you.

3. Some lollipops or peppermint sticks to suck on between contractions if you find that your mouth has become dry from the rapid superficial breathing. Generally you will not be allowed to drink water during labor, though you might be given a little crushed ice or be allowed to rinse your mouth. A lollipop or peppermint stick will feel good and even give you a little sugar.

4. A washcloth or a small sponge. Your husband can wet the washcloth or sponge and refresh your face. He can even let you suck on the wet sponge a little when your mouth gets dry.

5. A chapstick. Your lips may become very dry in labor, and your lipstick is usually not greasy enough to

keep them well lubricated. A chapstick will feel good and also stay on longer than lipstick.

6. A small paper bag to breathe in in case you hyperventilate.

7. A small can of talcum powder to smooth the skin when you or your partner massages your abdomen or any other part of your body.

8. Tennis balls or a can of tennis balls for counter pressure, should you have back labor.

9. Cool pack or Scotch ice to freeze the lower back, also in case you have back labor.

10. Mouth spray to freshen the breath.

11. Anything else you feel like putting in for practical reasons, for fun, or as a "security blanket."

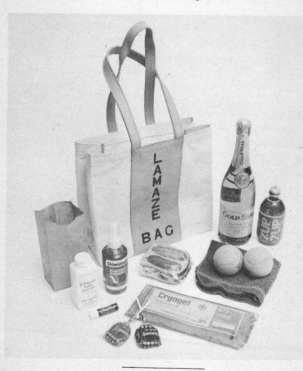

Do not put this Lamaze bag into your suitcase. Your suitcase will probably be taken immediately to the room that you will occupy once you have given birth. Carry it separately or let your husband bring it to you once he comes to the labor room.

ARRIVING
AT THE HOSPITAL

When you arrive at the hospital, you will usually have to go first to the admitting office. In some hospitals your partner can attend to the registration or you can even register weeks before you actually enter the hospital. Be sure to bring any necessary insurance cards along and perhaps your checkbook. Some hospitals ask for a deposit when you arrive if you haven't given them one at early registration. Of course they will always admit you, even if you've forgotten to bring a check, but it will cause less trouble at the time if you have it along.

Should you have a contraction while signing forms, don't hesitate to let the clerk wait until you have been able to control it with the appropriate breathing techniques and it has ended. Don't feel embarrassed when stopping in the middle of signing your name. After all, you are the one who is in labor at the moment, not the young woman who sits behind the desk!

You'll then be taken to the labor room, while your husband is asked to remain temporarily in the waiting room. In many hospitals your partner can stay with you when you first arrive at the hospital. It used to be that you were more or less immediately separated, once you entered the hospital, and reunited only after all examinations and "prepping" had been done. I think hospital authorities these days have come to realize that entering a hospital in labor is the first real crisis you have had to cope with. Any hospital stay is anxiety producing. But if your partner can stay with you, you will feel comforted and happy, not only to have him with you later in labor, but also at the beginning when you are being checked, examined and settled into the labor room.

You will undress completely and put on a hospital gown, a shorty which fastens in the back. This is not attractive but is quite practical. The nurse will ask you to give her a urine specimen, and she will take your temperature and your blood pressure. Then either your own doctor or a resident doctor will come and examine you. He will listen to the fetal heart, and check your heart and lungs. He will also ask you when your labor started, whether your membranes have broken, when you ate last, what you ate, etc. In many hospitals a nurse will take a blood sample to re-check your blood type, even though your doctor has done this previously at one of your prenatal visits. The doctor will then examine you internally, either rectally or vaginally. During this examination you should lie flat on your back, breathing deeply with your mouth open. This first internal examination is really most important for you. It will be the first signpost on your journey to the baby's birth. You will probably have been in labor at home for some hours, and no doubt will be eager to find out how much progress you've made so far. Your doctor may examine you during or between contractions. Be sure to ask the doctor how far you have effaced and dilated. Your own doctor will always communicate your progress to you, but don't be surprised if a resident physician seems reluctant to tell you this information. He doesn't know you personally and may not be aware that you are so well prepared for labor and delivery.

After this examination, a nurse will come and "prep" you. Recently a number of hospitals have started to change this procedure a little. They only clip the pubic hair and shave the anal hair. In some hospitals, neither "prep" nor enema are given anymore. You should tell your doctor beforehand that you prefer this kind of partial prepping, or no prepping at all.

It's a good idea to tell the nurse, before she starts to look after you, that you are going to use the Lamaze method. Be sure to ask her not to interrupt while you are using the breathing techniques, but explain that you will be glad to answer any questions as soon as the contraction is over. You will find the nurses most cooperative and helpful. They are usually fascinated at your being able to stay in control so efficiently.

The nurse will also give you an enema if the doctor has ordered one. During the enema breathe deeply, again through your mouth. In many hospitals you will be allowed to expel the enema on a toilet. In others you will be given a bedpan. Should you have to expel the enema on a bedpan, ask the nurse to place it on the edge of the bed and put a chair under the bed so that you can rest your feet and sit upright. Hospital beds are high and it is easy to place a chair under the bed. It is far more comfortable to expel in this way rather than having the pan placed in the middle of your bed. Stay on the toilet or bedpan for at least 20 minutes. If you don't give yourself enough time, you may find that with any subsequent contraction you will lose more stool and have to ask for another bedpan. Do not let anybody hurry you and continue with your breathing techniques whenever you have a contraction.

Now you are ready to ask the nurse to call your partner. (If you know beforehand that your partner cannot stay with you during this preliminary period, tell him ahead of time that the waiting period while you are being examined and "prepped" may be from 45 minutes to one hour. This is important for him to know, since an hour may seem a very long time to him. He may worry unduly or be afraid that he has been forgotten.)

Again, remind your partner to bring a sandwich or some cookies to eat in the hospital. He may get very hungry during your labor and it may be at night when all the coffee shops are closed. Or he may feel that he does not want to leave you alone to get a snack, even for half an hour. Alas, no matter how hungry you may feel, no eating is permitted during labor!

Ask the nurse to roll your bed up to any angle that suits you. You will have to experiment a little. Don't hesitate to ask for another pillow should you need it. If there is no second pillow available, ask the nurse for a blanket which she can roll up or fold to put wherever you need support. Most women feel far more comfortable in an upright position. The breathing is easier this way, and psychologically you will feel far more in control of the situation. The only time you'll have to lie down is when the doctor examines you, or if he feels that a certain position will be better for your labor.

BREATHING WITH YOUR LABOR

Remember that no labor will follow an exact textbook pattern. There is simply no way to plan in advance what breathing you will use at any given time. The great advantage of the Lamaze method is that you have acquired techniques to use as your labor demands from moment to moment. Do not anticipate a strict pattern, but react to the sensations that you feel at the time. Every labor is different from all others; it is up to you to adjust to your labor as it occurs. However, here are some fundamental rules to keep in mind:

1. Do not start any controlled breathing until you feel the absolute need for it.

2. Stay with the slow chest breathing as long as you can. It's much less fatiguing than the shallow, rapid breathing.

3. If you feel contractions in your back, ask your partner or the nurse to put pressure on your lower spine. You can massage or put pressure on yourself if necessary. Change positions to alleviate the discomfort of back labor by:

a. Sitting upright, leaning slightly forward so that the weight of the baby falls forward.

b. Lying on your side, placing the upper knee in front of the lower one. Place a pillow under the upper knee so that there is no strain on your thigh muscles.

c. Using the knee-chest position to take the pressure off your back.

d. Kneeling and leaning against the raised head of the bed.

4. Ask your partner to help you stay well relaxed. He must remind you to release your arms, legs, or shoulders or face whenever they get tense. You'll find that your homework pays off well here and that you will obey his commands automatically. This will give you both a feeling of doing a difficult job together.

5. Ask your partner to time the contractions and call out the intervals, 15 . . . 30 . . . 45 seconds. This will define and circumscribe the contractions. Once he calls out 45 seconds, you will know that the contraction will not go on much longer. Your beginning cleansing breath will be your husband's cue that the contraction has started. Occasionally it will be difficult for you to know exactly when the contraction has started. Your partner can help you in this case by putting his hand on the fundus, at the top of your uterus. He will usually be able to feel the tightening of the uterus with his fingers before you feel the actual sensation. He can then call out "Now!" and you can follow this command with your cleansing breath and breathing technique. Your partner should encourage and praise you, watching to see that you perform well. We all need encouragement, love and support during labor, especially when we are awake and actively participating in childbirth.

Frequently a fetal monitor is used either externally or internally on you almost as soon as you enter the hospital. This valuable machine monitors the fetal heartbeat, even during contractions, and at the same time shows the intensity of the uterine contractions on a paper on which a pen shows the curve pattern of the contraction. The external monitor is attached to your abdomen by two wide, elastic stockinette belts. This may make effleurage difficult, though you could confine the massage to the lower abdomen, where it is probably most beneficial anyway. The internal monitor will be attached by means of a small electrode to the presenting part of the baby, once the membranes have ruptured.

I would like to include a few words about the fetal monitor here. It is an electronic machine which assures a great safety factor for the baby during labor, as it points into the directions the staff should look if fetal heart irregularities occur.

THE FETAL MONITOR

The machine is invaluable for high-risk mothers or babies. If it is used, even though you may not be a high-risk mother, use it as an added indicator—almost like using biofeedback—to recognize the beginning, strength and end of a contraction. This makes it possible to stay with contractions, catch them on time with breathing techniques, in short, ride the waves. You will be able to watch a paper emerge from the monitor and follow the pen that is drawing the exact curve of your uterine contraction. In fact, you will find that the machine registers your contractions before you are actually aware of them.

It's important that you urinate whenever necessary during the first stage of labor. A large accumulation of urine may become quite uncomfortable and a full bladder takes up precious space in the abdominal cavity. You may find it a little difficult to urinate if the bladder is too full or if the uterus presses on it more and more as the baby descends. If you've had no medication, your husband can help you to the bathroom. If, however, you have had some sedation, ask the nurse for a bedpan.

Your doctor will examine you periodically during labor to determine what progress has been made. Always remember to ask your doctor about your progress after each examination. If he tells you how many centimeters you have dilated, it will give you a rough idea of how far along you've come. From time to time a nurse will listen to the fetal heart or watch the fetal monitor and take your blood pressure. This listening is important, as it is the only way the doctor and nurse can keep in touch with your baby during labor, and be sure that all is well.

THE USE OF MEDICATION

If at any time you should feel the need for medication or sedation, don't hesitate to ask for it. Your doctor will be happy to give you as much relief as he considers medically safe. If he himself suggests medication, he undoubtedly has good reasons for his decision, and I am sure he will explain and discuss them with you.

You've had many months during your prenatal visits to the doctor to discuss your and your partner's active participation in the birth of your child. Any medication he may give you will be necessary to insure both the health of your baby and your own safety. Even if you cannot be awake for the birth of your baby, your control and cooperation will help you cope with labor with less analgesia or anesthesia than you would ordinarily need.

BEGINNING TO PUSH

If you are expecting your first baby, you will probably begin the second stage of labor, or expulsion of the baby, in the labor room. As I have emphasized before, you must not push until the doctor has given you permission to push. If you have forgotten how to push, let your husband supervise you. You will probably find that after one or two pushing contractions you will be able to follow the instructions that you have been given. Do not forget to take your pillows to the delivery room so that your head and back can be raised on the delivery table.

It is generally assumed that every woman will have an overwhelming urge to push once she is fully dilated. This is not always so. The majority of women do feel the strong expulsive urge; I have found that the urge to push varies in intensity from woman to woman. There are also some women who never feel any urge whatsoever. The latter may be due to the position or the rotation of the baby. Should you be one of those who does not feel the urge to push and your doctor tells you to push with the next contraction, don't argue, "But I don't feel like it yet." Accept your physician's orders at the time without questioning, and use the pushing technique with the next contraction regardless of whether you feel like it or not.

In the delivery room, your partner will have to wear a cap, gown and mask. He will be told to stand next to your head and not to move from there unless he is asked to do so by your physician. You will be draped, and must remember to keep your hands firmly on the handles or stirrups. Remember, do not touch any of the sterile sheets. Before you start to push on the delivery table, the nurse will pour some disinfectant over your pubic area. This will feel icy cold, but it is actually quite a refreshing surprise!

YOUR BABY ARRIVES!

Your doctor will give you the command to push, once you are on the table. Be sure to pant or blow out whenever he asks you to stop pushing. This allows the doctor time to ease the baby along; he helps deliver the head and shoulders, receiving the rest of the baby's body, which then slips out easily into his hands.

And so you have given birth to your baby! Your doctor will hold the baby up by its feet in order to drain the mucus from its mouth and nose. At this point your baby will cry heartily.

Babies do not come out looking washed and immaculate. Your baby will be wet and wrinkled. It will have patches of a whitish cream all over its body, which is the protective coating, or "vernix," which the baby had while growing in your uterus, and it will look bluish gray for a few seconds before it starts to cry and the color of its skin changes to pink. Black babies will look very light when born. This pigmentation occurs gradually.

Your doctor will then put the baby on your abdomen. Remember, this is the sterile area, therefore an excellent place to put the baby while the umbilical cord is clamped and cut. But keep your hands under the drapes. You will have to wait just a little longer before you are allowed to hold your child.

Once the cord has been cut—which does not hurt either you or the baby—the nurse will wrap it in a warm blanket and put it into a bassinette, which is slightly tilted to help the baby expel more mucus and make breathing easier. The nurse will put a plastic identification band on the baby and on you. Your fingerprints may be taken and possibly the baby's footprints. A few drops of silver nitrate may be put into the baby's eyes, or the baby may be given a penicillin shot instead.

A number of physicians and midwives adopt some of Dr. Leboyer's ideas these days. Also, many couples are asking that Leboyer's approach, i.e., "the baby is a person," be used. Lights are dimmed in the delivery room, except for a spotlight on the mother's pelvic floor. The baby stays for a longer period on the mother's abdomen so that she can touch it gently, rub its back and establish eye contact with her child.

At this point you will be given an injection of a hormone which helps expel the placenta, contract the uterus and prevent excessive bleeding. In the meantime, you may have another contraction. The doctor will feel your uterus and decide that it is time for you to "express" the placenta (our third stage of labor). Be sure to help the doctor with another good push to expel the placenta. The doctor will assist you by putting gentle pressure on your abdomen. It will take no more than two to three minutes to expel the placenta. Now your hard work is over.

If he has performed an episiotomy, your doctor will clean you up and perform "the repair" or stitching. While he is doing this ask to hold your baby. Frequently you'll get to hold and talk to it while your doctor does the repair. Your husband will also hold and touch the baby and help you put the baby to your breast should you desire to nurse it right there and then.

Your partner's place is always next to you, so that he can talk to you, helping to raise your head and shoulders when you push. Under no circumstances should he look over the doctor's shoulder unless he is actually asked to come to the doctor's side.

AFTER YOU'VE GIVEN BIRTH

For about two hours after you have given birth, a nurse will watch you closely. She will massage your abdomen from time to time to make sure that your uterus remains firm. Occasionally the nurse will show you how to massage your abdomen yourself.

Now you will be taken back to your own bed in your own room. You will probably feel fantastically elated! You may not be able to sleep much the first night after you've given birth. You'll be proud of your baby and of yourself, of your husband and of your ability to have functioned so well.

However, there is still some immediate work ahead of you. Do not forget to do your pelvic floor contractions; they will speed your recovery. Also you *will* experience some slight continued contractions, which are a good sign that your uterus is healing and contracting again to its original size. These contractions after childbirth will be more pronounced if this was your second, third or fourth delivery, since it becomes more difficult for the muscles to regain their original tone. You are also likely to feel them when you nurse your baby.

Please remember that these contractions occur for a very good reason: to get your uterus back to its usual size. They are a sign of a speedy recovery.

And so you have given birth to your baby. You have joined all the thousands of mothers and fathers who have trained themselves to give birth actively instead of passively, and you have prepared yourself diligently for the first step on the road to successful parenthood.

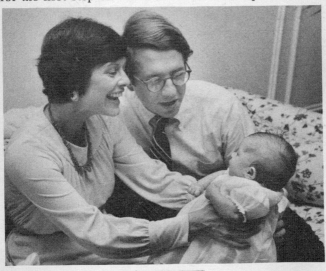

A
MOTHER'S
REPORT

BY PHYLIS FEINSTEIN

*A personal, moment-by-moment account
by a young woman, prepared with the
Lamaze method, of her first childbirth*

The beginning of my labor was less than auspicious. My first indication that the baby would be born this year yet occurred Tuesday around 1:30 P.M. when my mucous plug came out. No contractions, no showing . . . nothing.

All afternoon I waited. About once every half hour I'd get a tiny tweak in my pelvic area, but it was so short and inconsequential that I'm still not sure I didn't wish it into existence. I called Richard, my husband, a dozen times during the course of the day to tell him not to come home yet. However, I also informed him it could happen any minute.

For some reason every appliance in our house got serviced that Tuesday. And so the washing machine got its new grounding wire, the dryer a new catch, etc. I was busy answering the door all afternoon, feeling fine—if a little apprehensive. Checking my preparation for when labor would begin, I found a half bowl of Jello in the refrigerator (if I should get hungry during the earliest stages), a container of stew in the freezer (for Richard to take to the hospital in a wide-mouthed thermos in case he got hungry), my luggage packed and my Lamaze goodie bag complete.

About the goodie bag: I had decided to make it particularly nice, figuring that at the time I would need it, any pleasantry would help. And so the bag itself was not an ordinary brown, dull grocery model. This was a slick-papered pink (prophetic) bag, the kind lazy gift-givers use instead of fancy wrapping paper on the outside of presents. Inside was a brand-new flowered washcloth—blue (unprophetic)—my favorite talc (we used practically the entire can), chap-stick, some fancy lollipops, and the three-dollar-wonder of a clock I used to time my breathing exercises. The clock has a cracked face, no minute hand, but the niftiest second hand. I was confidently prepared . . . until 3:00 A.M. Wednesday morning, when the first real contraction lifted me out of a deep sleep. I bolted from my warm bed groaning, "My God, I've got back labor." Naturally this woke Richard, and for the next half hour all the careful planning, the long, intellectual discussions about not panicking were forgotten.

We were both in a maddening state of hysteria. I couldn't face having back labor.

Richard couldn't face that I was in labor and, after assuring me labor doesn't start this way, he said in his most condescending tone, "Obviously, you're constipated." Then he added, "Gee, I'm starving," and dove into the refrigerator.

Meanwhile I sat on a kitchen stool, effleuraging like mad, breathing properly and quietly swearing alternately at back labor and at my husband. I soon checked my contractions at five-minute intervals, when I mustered, "Richard, you'd better call the doctor."

Richard acquiesced. In his Cary Grant manner he began the conversation suavely, "Hello, Doctor. How are you?" (At 3:00 in the morning!) "Yes, this is Richard Feinstein. Phylis *thinks* she's in labor. Every five minutes. Clock them for another half hour and if they are steady call back? Call back anyway? O.K."

By fifteen minutes later the contractions were coming every four minutes. We called our doctor again and were told to come nearer the hospital (we live half an hour away) and wait a bit at my cousin's, who lives only a block from the hospital. We forgot Richard's stew. But before we left he ate my Jello. And while I dressed he managed to brew some tea and pack some fruit for the trip. By this time I had hold of myself, and found the ride on the parkway uneventful. Richard concentrated on the road and I on my contractions. I cracked open the package of lollipops and lapped away when my mouth became dry. (First mistake: Don't buy sweet pops. The smaller, sourer ones are much better.)

I had beside me two pillows I'd grabbed just in case the hospital was short-stocked. It proved to be good thinking!

We arrived at my cousin's at 4:00 A.M. The door was opened by two sleepy and excited relatives. Now my contractions were two minutes apart. Another call to the doctor and we were off to the hospital at last. We entered, Richard carrying my goodie bag and his box lunch and I clutching my pillows and sucking my too-sweet lollipop. We were quite a pair.

An o.b. nurse was sent down to accompany me to the maternity floor. In the elevator she looked me up and down, taking in my pillows and lollipop.

"Why those?" She pointed.

I said, "Pillows for back support. Pops for dry mouth."

Off the elevator she headed me toward a room I shared with three other ladies. I readied for bed and, in between shallow breathing techniques, I asked a nurse to roll up my bed.

She did, muttering, "Everyone lies down for labor, you sit like a tailor sewing."

She left as Richard returned from signing me in. He dismantled the bag, placing the talc, washcloth, chapstick and lollies close by. The doctor arrived, followed by a blonde bulldozer of a nurse. She looked at Richard and said, "Better you wait in the solarium. Better still wait downstairs till it's over." In unison Richard and I said, "No, he's going to stay." The nurse aimed her attack at the doctor. "You know the rules—husbands stay only by special permission of the hospital president."

"Fine," said Dr. H. "Call Harvey."

She: "Harvey" (the name stuck in her throat) "doesn't like being called at 4:30 A.M."

Dr. H.: "He's been called before. Let's talk about this."

And they stepped around my tent and left the room. Richard timed my contractions; I rubbed my belly.

Ten minutes later, Dr. H. came back and broke my water. I was put on a movable table and taken to a private room, where Richard and I spent the entire labor.

We were finally settled and ready for action. For the first time I had a chance to evaluate what was happening inside me. I wasn't having true back labor because, Dr. H. assured me, the baby was not in a posterior position. The contractions began at the back, reached their peak about three inches below my navel and then spread in both directions toward my hips as they subsided. I was breathing as directed in the second stage of the first part of labor (dilation)—cleansing breath, slow breath, acceleration as the contraction built and then regaining a slow pace as it lessened. The doctor examined me at 5:30 and told us the good news. I was 5½ centimeters dilated. Richard was busy indeed sprinkling on talc, pouring water on my tongue and lips, applying chapstick. I would point and he would do. In between such activities he sat on the chair near the bed and drew me (perhaps the first portrait of a pregnant Lamaze in labor) or surreptitiously snitched a grape from his lunch pail. The doctor left the room, promising to return in an hour. Everything was concentrated on my work. And it *was* work.

The analogy comparing the contraction control of riding a wave is excellent. And once I caught the "wave" and rode it until it broke quietly on the shores of my conscious being, I smiled. *Smiled* during labor. When I think of pain I think of something sharper, something stabbing. Nothing like that kind of pain happened. I could feel what seemed to be a regular agonizing stretching, very uncomfortable, but with all my breathing and concentration, it was easily bearable! Dr. H. came back at 6:30 and said I was doing fine.

At 7:00 he examined me. The news—8 to 8½ centimeters. I was in transition and I didn't even know it! Contractions were coming at exactly one minute, forty-five seconds. "How much longer?" I hoarsely whispered.

"About two and a half hours." Dr. H. replied. He was off by fourteen minutes!

The new shift of nurses arrived at 7:00. As fate would have it they were the same wonderful group that showed me around the maternity floor a month earlier. What a cheering section they turned out to be! They breathed with me, came in between their duties to encourage me, were in the delivery room when Amanda was born. Dr. H. never left the room from 7:00 on. Just letting us know that he was very much a part of what was going on by being there. The only time he asked me if I wanted any medication was about 4:30 A.M. He said it to reassure me, I guess. But he never offered it again. Even when the going got tough during the last stage of transition. After the birth, I asked why he never again mentioned it. His answer: "Who needed it?"

By 8:00 I was 9½ centimeters and fagged out. I wanted to push, but Dr. H. said not yet. I wanted to push very badly. I lost my breathing, grabbed for Richard's and Dr. H's hands, blew out all my good oxygen and squeezed their hands. "It's time," I moaned. Dr. H's examination showed I was wrong. The cervix had just a little left to dilate, enough to make a difference between pushing uselessly and productive expulsion. Meanwhile Richard got me on the road to breathing properly by forcing me to listen to him do it. Thirty minutes later came the word—*push!* They rolled down the bed. I got into position (after Richard reminded me to get into position) and I pushed. Erroneously I thought three good pushes and out would come baby. Ha!

The hardest part, for me, was the expulsion. It hurt and I was tired. "No more pushing," I groaned, just as the doctor said, "Come here, Richard—here comes your baby's head and the hair's black." Rich rushed around the bed. Then I grinned and said, "Who's tired?" I wanted to push more than anything else in the world.

They took us to the delivery room. Dr. H. administered a local for the episiotomy. What seemed like five pushes—good ones—and then minutes later the doctor lifted up the biggest, most beautiful girl baby I've ever seen: 8 pounds, 2 ounces, 21 inches of Lamaze testimonial.

I don't know words to describe it.

A
FATHER'S
REPORT

BY PATRICK CASEY

*The role of the husband is crucial
throughout labor and delivery; here
is one man's report of his experience*

The birth of our first child had been an unpleasant experience. My wife had no real idea of what to expect when those first contractions came four years ago. She was surprised, frightened and extremely uncomfortable. Neither of us had any notion that childbirth could be such a harrowing ordeal. After a few moments of desperate handholding I was asked to leave the hospital room; she was heavily medicated and, at the end of several hours of anxiety and confusion, I was informed that our first son had arrived. Happily, he was a fine, healthy baby, but the experience was so distressing that for a long time Marilyn would not consider going through the whole thing again.

Eventually we did decide to have another child. About the same time Marilyn become pregnant again a friend told us about a marvelous new technique of childbirth called the Lamaze Method. A clear idea of what happens physically during labor and delivery, a few exercises to prepare the body, a system of breathing to alleviate discomfort during contractions and a supporting role for the husband—it sounded practical, worth investigating. Certainly we wanted to do something to avoid another traumatic experience, so we went to an obstetrician who encouraged the Lamaze Method and enrolled in the six-lesson course.

Those weekly sessions were really quite marvelous. Not only did they lift the traditional veil of mystery about childbirth by simply explaining what was going to happen and how to prepare for it, but they helped eliminate any nervous apprehension about the whole event. By creating a warm atmosphere of rational discussion, and by giving us specific exercises and techniques to practice together, the classes gradually dispelled our anxieties. We aired our questions with the other four couples in the class; we worked together at home; we arranged with the doctor and hospital that I be allowed to be with Marilyn in the labor and delivery room. The whole thing became a happy collaboration, something we were preparing for as husband and wife.

The first contractions came at about 3:00 A.M. a few days after the anticipated date of delivery. Marilyn woke me at 3:30, announcing that she had been having what "could be real contractions" for half an hour. By 4 A.M. I was calling Dr. A. to report regular mild contractions about five minutes apart. We knew that a second baby usually comes faster than the first, but we were surprised to hear him tell us to get down to the hospital as quickly as we could. Marilyn's suitcase and the little Lamaze bag had both been carefully packed weeks before. Without further delay we hopped in a cab.

Marilyn's water hadn't broken yet—the first thing that happened when Jonathan was born—but as we sped toward the hospital her contractions continued to be definite and regular. I suggested that she begin the first breathing technique, but she refused, reminding me that we had been taught to wait until it was absolutely necessary. At 4:30 we pulled up to the night entrance of the hospital.

We had registered and left a deposit with the hospital a month before, so we went straight up to the fourth-floor delivery area where Dr. A. was already waiting. In a wonderfully paternal manner he took Marilyn into the labor room to be dressed and examined while I changed into regulation sterile-white shirt and pants next door. About ten minutes later I joined Marilyn in the labor room, where one pillow was under her head and another under her knees. She told me that she was already 5 centimeters dilated and would allegedly have the baby within the hour. It was now 4:45 A.M. We were both terribly excited as she began doing the accelerated breathing. I made myself useful by powdering her abdomen and giving her a lollipop to suck on between contractions. Marilyn laughed at my hospital get-up. She thought it would be a girl. I was noncommittal.

A friendly nurse bustled in and out, while a resident technician took a sample of blood. The contractions had been mild and relatively close together, but now were getting slightly stronger and more difficult to control. It was exactly like our practice at home: Marilyn breathed and concentrated on a spot across the little room, while I called off fifteen-second intervals of the contraction.

At 5:10 things quickened; Marilyn began having really strong contractions. Immediately we shifted into the rapid breathing and blowing method of breathing. The doctor came in, made a quick examination and called for the nurse; we were going into the delivery room! I grabbed two pillows and tried to keep up with the rolling table, while fitting on my cap and face mask. The nurse laughed at me as I trotted along, dropping a pillow every three feet, but dauntlessly following everyone into the delivery room where Marilyn was already being transferred to the table. Now the contractions were quite intense and she really had to hold back the urge to push and force herself to concentrate on breathing.

The atmosphere in the delivery room was something like a congenial clubhouse. I was introduced to the anesthesiologist ("He's here just in case we need any medication.") and to the two nurses who were performing little chores about the room with towels and instruments. The baby's head was about to show, the doctor told us, and with the next contraction he would break the membranes and Marilyn could at last begin to push. I mopped her brow, which really wasn't at all necessary, and tried to keep busy arranging the pillows beneath her head.

"Ready," Dr. A. said quietly, as Marilyn took her two deep breaths, held the third and pushed. A fierce growl-like noise filled the room as she bared her teeth, straining down and out, gripping the metal bars of the table. I think she must have been oblivious to everything else in the room, so powerful was her concentration and determination. A gush of water shot across the room.

"Good!" the doctor said, ". . . and again . . ."

The incredible noise she made! And the strength of her face. It was like watching some legendary hero perform a Herculean triumph, toppling a temple, overthrowing a false god, defeating an enemy.

"Very good! Come and look—you can see the baby's hair."

I rushed to peer over the doctor's shoulder. There was the top of the baby's head, plastered with what looked then like dark hair.

Marilyn gave a faint smile and prepared to push again. At this point the doctor gave Marilyn an injection of local anesthetic and made an incision, painlessly, to enlarge the opening. One last push and I saw the head come completely out. Dr. A. worked his hand under the shoulder and in a second the whole child slid easily into the world.

"It's a boy!" the anesthesiologist said, first to notice from his vantage point at Marilyn's head. "The time is 5:37."

It was indeed a boy, looking quite wrinkled and angry. Being a naturally anxious sort, I was relieved to note that he had only one head, two arms, two legs, etc. His skin had a bluish tinge, as he hung from the doctor's grip, and his little body was tense. The umbilical cord ran from his navel to the placenta, which had not yet been expelled. The cord was clamped and cut, while I fretted about his lifeless appearance. The doctor then gave him a slap on the soles of his feet. (Apparently, spanking the bottom is only for the movies.) There was a gurgle deep in the baby's throat, in another second a faint cry, and then a series of lusty yells and wails. He was really alive—very much so!

Dr. A. ordered another short push to expel the placenta, and in no time at all he had stitched up the episiotomy. In the meantime, we could not take our eyes off little Peter Nicholas (for that was to be his name), who was getting pinker and pinker in the glass box he had been placed in next to the delivery table. We could see now that what I had thought was dark hair was really wet red hair, exactly the same shade as his mother's and brother's.

Then we were left quite alone. The anesthesiologist packed up his tanks and left. The nurses were in and out, and the doctor went off to see about another woman who had arrived in labor.

It was the proudest, happiest moment of our lives. Here was our new son, after only two hours of mild labor and absolutely no medication whatsoever, not even an aspirin! The difference between this and our first childbirth was miraculous. Marilyn had used the Lamaze Method to perfection. The method had given us calmness with which we both approached the event, confidence with which we were able to cope with each succeeding stage, joy in doing all this together, and this ultimate, happy reward.

ABOUT THE AUTHOR

ELISABETH BING was born in Berlin, Germany, of a distinguished scientific family. She was trained as a physical therapist in London, England, and came to New York in 1949. She worked under Dr. Alan Guttmacher in the Childbirth Education Program at the Mt. Sinai Hosital from 1952 until 1960. Elisabeth Bing became one of the co-founders of the American Society for Psychoprophylaxis in Obstetrics, Inc. in 1960. Since then she has continued her hospital work at the Flower and Fifth Avenue hospitals as instructor in childbirth education for the department of obstetrics and gynecology of the N.Y. Medical College. While continuing her hospital work, Ms. Bing has trained thousands of expectant parents in her own private classes. She has traveled widely all over the U.S. and Europe, giving workshops, lecturing and holding seminars in many colleges, hospitals and communities.

Bantam Book Catalog

It lists over a thousand money-saving bestsellers originally priced from $3.75 to $15.00 —bestsellers that are yours now for as little as 60¢ to $2.95!

The catalog gives you a great opportunity to build your own private library at huge savings!

So don't delay any longer—send us your name and address and 25¢ (to help defray postage and handling costs).

About this book

This book is divided into five sections.

The essence of Eastern Canada
pages 6–19
Introduction; Features; Food and drink; Short break including the 10 Essentials

Planning pages 20–33
Before you go; Getting there; Getting around; Being there

Best places to see pages 34–55
The unmissable highlights of any visit to Eastern Canada

Best things to do pages 56–79
Good places to have lunch; train and boat trips; stunning views and more

Exploring pages 80–186
The best places to visit in Eastern Canada, organized by area

♛ to ♛♛♛♛ denotes AAA rating

Maps
All map references are to the maps on the covers. For example, Ottawa has the reference ✚ 9D – indicating the grid square in which it is to be found.

Admission prices
Inexpensive (under Can$6)
Moderate (Can$6–$12)
Expensive (over Can$12)

Hotel prices
Per room per night:
$ budget (under Can$75)
$$ moderate (Can$75–$150)
$$$ expensive to luxury (over Can$150)

Restaurant prices
Price for a three-course meal per person without drinks:
$ budget (under Can$25)
$$ moderate (Can$25–$40)
$$$ expensive (over Can$40)

Contents

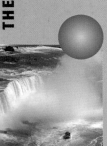
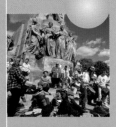
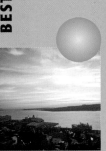

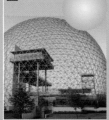
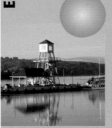

The essence of...

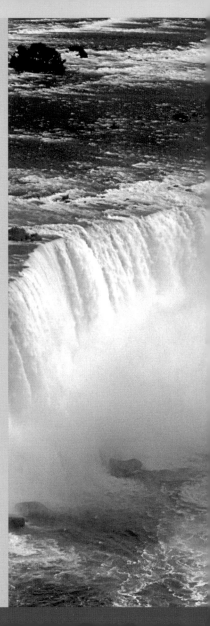

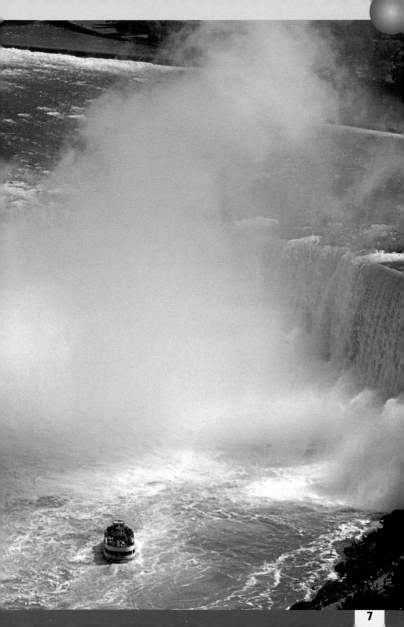

Eastern Canada is huge, so don't try to see it all in one go. Instead, include a little of everything during your trip. The Atlantic coast is an essential destination, from the intriguing lifestyle of Newfoundland to the wonderful scenery of Cape Breton and glorious New Brunswick beaches. Inland are more natural beauties: the vast Great Lakes and the popular Niagara Falls.

Eastern Canada also has sophisticated cities. Toronto has fine modern architecture, Montréal abounds in splendid restaurants, Ottawa offers great museums and Québec has a stunning site and a resolutely French face. In all, there's something here for everyone.

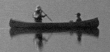

features

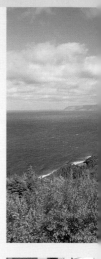

Eastern Canada is a land of great variety. Nowhere is this more true than in the Atlantic provinces, where you can experience the Bay of Fundy and its dramatic tides, the wild Atlantic coast of Nova Scotia, spectacular Cape Breton, the tranquil beauty of Prince Edward Island and the rugged landscapes of Newfoundland.

The natural beauty of Eastern Canada is complemented by vibrant cities and towns, among them Montréal and Toronto, each one unique in character and charm.

Finally, despite the crowds, don't miss standing on the brink of Niagara Falls watching all that water endlessly falling over the rock edge.

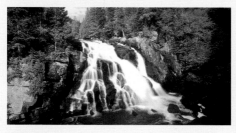

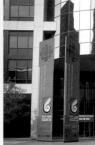

GEOGRAPHY

● Most of Ontario, Québec and Labrador are part of the Canadian Shield, rich in minerals, covered with forest and traversed by fast-flowing rivers.

● The five Great Lakes cover 244,000sq km (more than 94,000sq miles). The deepest is Lake Superior, with a maximum depth of 406m (1,332ft).

● The St. Lawrence River is Eastern Canada's major waterway. Although it is only 1,223km (760 miles) long, its drainage basin covers nearly 518,000sq km (200,000sq miles).

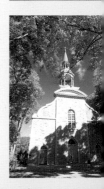

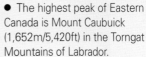

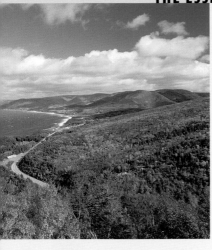

● The highest peak of Eastern Canada is Mount Caubuick (1,652m/5,420ft) in the Torngat Mountains of Labrador.
● Newfoundland and Labrador's craggy coastline stretches for around 9,900km (6,152 miles).

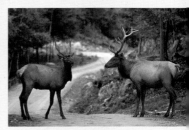

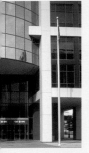

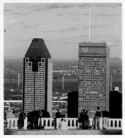

ANIMAL LIFE
● The forests are the domain of many animals including moose, deer, beaver and a variety of bears. The north also has caribou.
● Canada geese are all over the region. They are particularly prominent during migration, when they fly in vast V-shaped formations.

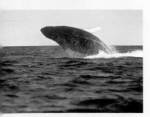

● Several types of whales can be seen around the coast of Nova Scotia and New Brunswick's Bay of Fundy, and in the St. Lawrence near the mouth of the Saguenay every summer (► 54–55).

SPORTS AND LEISURE
● Hockey is the national obsession, and it's played on ice of course!
● The fabulous natural countryside of Eastern Canada is ideal for outdoor activities such as camping, canoeing, hiking and fishing, and skiing, skating and snowmobiling in winter.

food & drink

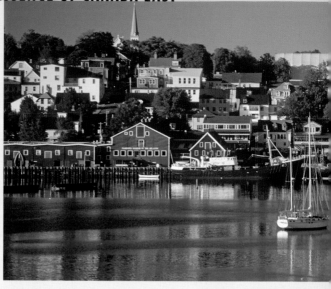

ATLANTIC PROVINCES

Not surprisingly for a region so closely connected with the sea, there is seafood galore here: large, luscious Malpeque oysters from Prince Edward Island (PEI); tender Digby scallops from Nova Scotia; and fat red lobsters from New Brunswick (Shediac is "the lobster capital of the world") and also from PEI, where attendance at a community lobster supper is *de rigueur*. In New Brunswick, the Atlantic salmon is wonderful; Oven Head, near St. Andrews-by-the-Sea, is a great place to buy it smoked.

In Newfoundland, fish and *brewis* (salt codfish and seabiscuit) is a favorite dish, while for dessert you could try figgy duff, a steaming-hot raisin pudding. In the Acadian areas, chicken *fricot* (hearty

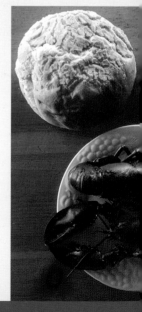

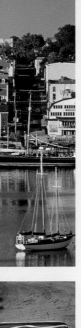

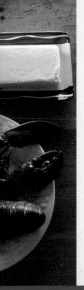

chicken soup) will warm you up, or try *poutine rappé* (potato dumpling with salt pork).

In Halifax, Alexander Keith's India pale ale is distinctly hoppy in flavor. Drink it with Solomon Grundy (marinated herring – a touch salty), or swig it down with fiddleheads, the tender curled ends of ferns, lightly boiled and slathered in butter. For a sweet treat, buy chocolates from Chocolatier Ganong in St. Stephen, New Brunswick, widely available in stores.

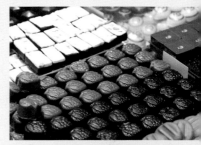

QUÉBEC

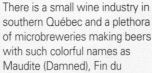

There is a small wine industry in southern Québec and a plethora of microbreweries making beers with such colorful names as Maudite (Damned), Fin du Monde (End of the World) and Eau Bénite (Holy Water). As an aperitif or after-dinner drink, try Sortilège, made from maple syrup and Canadian whisky, or Chicoutai, made from cloudberries.

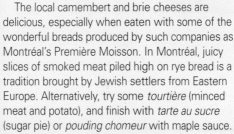

The local camembert and brie cheeses are delicious, especially when eaten with some of the wonderful breads produced by such companies as Montréal's Première Moisson. In Montréal, juicy slices of smoked meat piled high on rye bread is a tradition brought by Jewish settlers from Eastern Europe. Alternatively, try some *tourtière* (minced meat and potato), and finish with *tarte au sucre* (sugar pie) or *pouding chomeur* with maple sauce.

Apples grown in the Rougemont area are used to make alcoholic ciders, apple vinegars and even iced

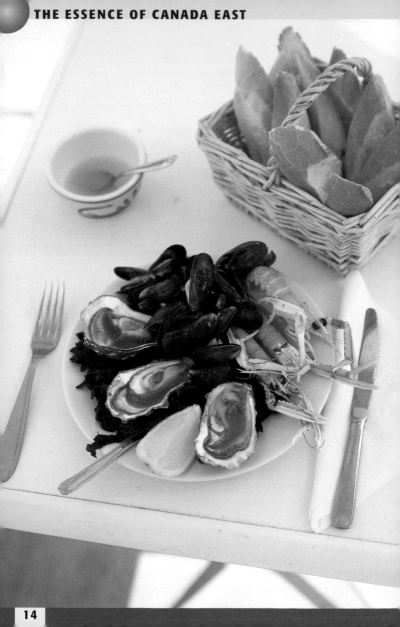

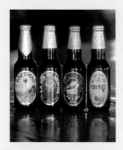

cider. The latter is delicious with foie gras, a side product of the ducks raised around Brome Lake, where thinly sliced *magret de canard* (duck breast) is a specialty. On Île d'Orléans, the Domaine Steinbach is one of several places in Québec making wonderful mustards.

In spring, a visit to a *cabane à sucre* (sugar shack) is fun. Celebrate the end of winter like a local by pouring maple syrup over everything – ham, beans, eggs, pancakes and so on. Wash it all down with a glass of caribou (a lethal mixture of brandy, vodka, sherry and port) or a kir (white wine and crème de cassis). And don't forget to try some maple taffy – hot maple syrup poured onto the snow and then eaten off a stick.

Popular with Québecois teenagers, and known as *poutine,* is a cholesterol-heavy mixture of French fries, cheese curds and gravy. You can even get the dish at McDonald's, and it has spread to the other eastern provinces too.

ONTARIO

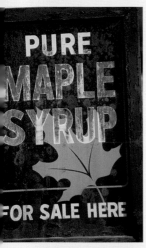

The Niagara peninsula is a famous wine-making area that is also known for its ice wine, made with grapes that have frozen on the vine. It is quite sweet and rather expensive. There's lots of fresh produce here too – peaches, cherries, apricots and so on – as well as delicious jams.

Toronto has excellent restaurants known for their "fusion cuisine," but it's also a center for ethnic food from every corner of the world. Try visiting Kensington Market on a Saturday (▶ 162–163) or the St. Lawrence Market in Toronto for a peameal bacon sandwich (▶ 184). Canadian Club Whisky has been made in Walkerville (Windsor) for more than 150 years. It's lighter than scotch, smoother than bourbon, and is a great accompaniment to Canadian cheddar cheese made in Ingersoll.

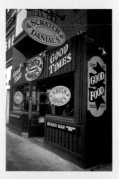

short break

If you only have a short time to visit Eastern Canada and would like to take home some unforgettable memories try doing something that captures the real flavor of the region. The following suggestions feature classic sights and experiences that won't cost very much and will make your visit very special.

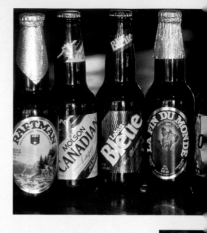

● **Drive the Cabot Trail** (➤ 70) through the Cape Breton Highlands National Park (➤ 38–39) to experience the most breathtaking scenery on one of the most beautiful islands in the world.

● **Take the boat trip** into Western Brook Pond in Gros Morne National Park (➤ 95) to wonder at this spectacular and deserted fjord, which is 16km (10 miles) long, 3km (2 miles) wide and 160m (525ft) deep.

● **Enjoy a lobster supper** on Prince Edward Island (➤ 100–101).

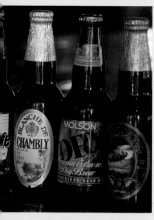

● **Picnic on the slopes of the Citadelle** in Québec City (➤ 127) on a summer evening and watch the sun set across the St. Lawrence River.

● **Order a beer** (or a *café au lait*, if it's early in the day) at one of the cafés on place Jacques Cartier (➤ 122) in Montréal and watch the world walk by, or be entertained by the street performers.

● **Take a jet-boat trip up the St. Lawrence** to the Lachine Rapids near Montréal and get soaked by the spray (or, for the adventurous, raft down the same rapids).

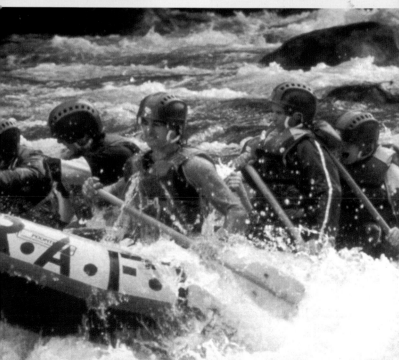

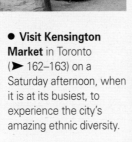

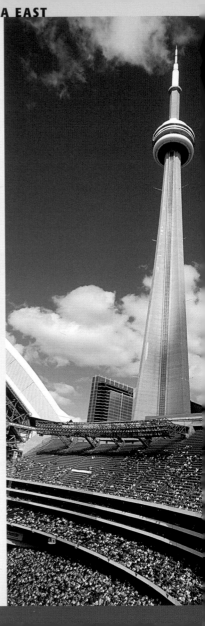

● **Visit Kensington Market** in Toronto (➤ 162–163) on a Saturday afternoon, when it is at its busiest, to experience the city's amazing ethnic diversity.

● **Go to the top of the CN Tower** (➤ 40–41) – after all, at 553.33m (1,815ft 5in), it is the world's tallest free-standing building!

● **Skate the length of the Rideau Canal** in Ottawa (➤ 157) in February, especially at the end of the day to watch the civil servants skating home from work as the sun sets.

● **Stand on the brink of the Niagara Falls** (➤ 44–45) and be mesmerized by the falling water. You may even forget the crowds – 14 million people visit the falls every year!

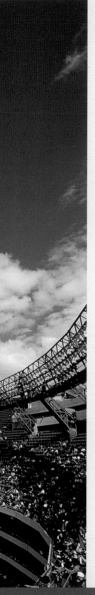

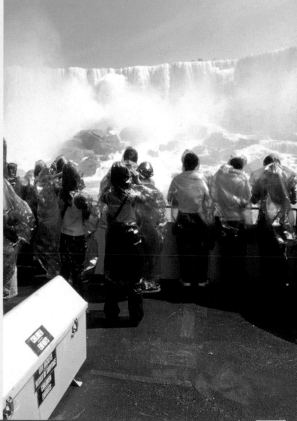

Planning

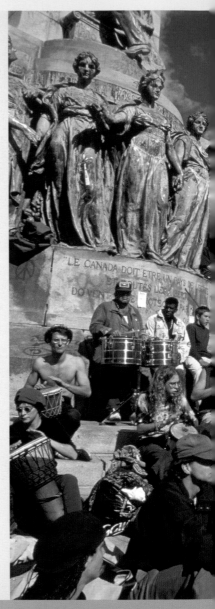

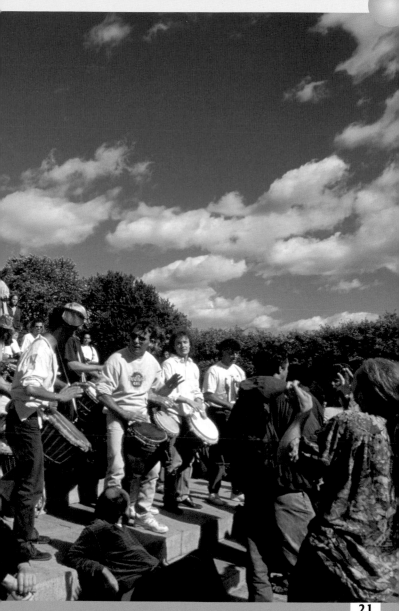

Before you go

WHEN TO GO

JAN	FEB	MAR	APR	MAY	JUN	JUL	AUG	SEP	OCT	NOV	DEC
-8°C	-7°C	-1°C	7°C	17°C	23°C	26°C	25°C	21°C	13°C	6°C	1°C
18°F	19°F	30°F	45°F	63°F	73°F	79°F	77°F	70°F	55°F	43°F	34°F

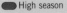
🔴 High season   🔵 Low season

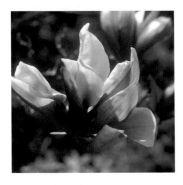

Mostly, summers are warm and can actually get hot – in southern Ontario temperatures often reach 30°C (86°F) and humidity makes these days uncomfortable. It's fresher in coastal areas, and can be just as warm, though rain and fog are often seen; coastal winters are often milder than in much of Canada, but all regions get a great deal of snow.

WHAT YOU NEED

● Required
○ Suggested
▲ Not required

Some countries require a passport to remain valid for a minimum period (usually at least six months) beyond the date of entry – contact their consulate or embassy or your travel agent for details.

	UK	Germany	USA	France	Spain
Passport (or other acceptable form of ID)	●	●	●	●	●
Visa (regulations can change – check before you travel)	▲	▲	▲	▲	▲
Onward or Return Ticket	○	○	○	○	○
Health Innoculations (tetanus and polio)	▲	▲	▲	▲	▲
Travel Insurance	○	○	○	○	○
Driving License (national)	●	●	●	●	●
Car Insurance Certificate	●	●	●	●	●
Car Registration Document	●	●	●	●	●

WEBSITES
- http://canada.gc.ca
- http://canadainternational.gc.ca
- www.pc.gc.ca
- www.canada.travel

TOURIST OFFICES
In the U.S.A. Canadian Tourism Commission, Yvonne Nichie (New York) ☎ 212/689-9307
Kristine Sigurdson (Los Angeles) ☎ 310/643-7768

In the U.K. Canadian Tourism Commission ✉ Visit Canada, PO Box 101, Chard TA20 9AR ☎ (0870) 380 0070

In Australia Canadian Tourism Commission ✉ Suite 105, Jones Bay Wharf, 26–32 Pirrama Road, Pyrmont, NSW 2009 ☎ (02) 9571 1665; fax: (02) 9571 1766

HEALTH INSURANCE
Visitors requiring treatment while in Canada must pay for it, which can be expensive. It is essential to take out health insurance. Make sure you keep all receipts to make a claim. Also ensure your coverage includes a "repatriation" clause in case no suitable treatment is available.

If you require dental help (expensive), ask at the reception desk of your hotel. Most hotels have a list of dentists.

TIME DIFFERENCES

Ottawa (EST)	New York	Los Angeles	London	Tokyo	Sydney
12 noon	12 noon	9AM	5PM	2AM	5AM

Eastern Canada has four different time zones. Most of Ontario and Québec observe Eastern Standard Time (EST). The most westerly part of Ontario observes Central Standard Time (EST -1). New Brunswick, Nova Scotia, Prince Edward Island, Labrador, and part of eastern Québec observe Atlantic Standard Time (EST +1). The island of Newfoundland observes Newfoundland Standard Time (1.5 hours ahead of EST). Daylight Saving Time (DST) is observed from mid-March to early November.

NATIONAL AND PROVINCIAL HOLIDAYS

Jan 1 *New Year's Day*
Mar 17 *St. Patrick's Day* (Newfoundland and Labrador)
Mar–Apr *Good Friday*
Mar–Apr *Easter Monday*
Apr 23 *St. George's Day* (Newfoundland and Labrador)
May (Mon closest to 24) *Victoria Day*
Jun 24 *St-Jean-Baptiste Day* (Québec)
Jun 24 *Discovery Day* (Newfoundland and Labrador)
Jul 1 *Canada Day*
Jul 12 *Orangeman's Day* (Newfoundland and Labrador)
Aug (1st Mon) *New Brunswick Day* (New Brunswick)
Aug (1st Mon) *Civic holiday* (Ontario)
Aug (1st Mon) *Natal Day* (Nova Scotia, except in Halifax, usually Jul or Aug)
Aug (1st Mon) *Natal Day* (PEI – by proclamation)
Aug *Regatta Day/civic holiday* (Newfoundland and Labrador – fixed by municipal council orders)
Sep (1st Mon) *Labour Day*
Oct (2nd Mon) *Thanksgiving* (note: this is not at the same time as American Thanksgiving)
Nov 11 *Remembrance Day* (not celebrated in Québec)
Dec 25 *Christmas Day*
Dec 26 *Boxing Day*

WHAT'S ON WHEN
Festival Nation
The festivals and events listed here are the best-known and most established in Eastern Canada, for example, Canada Day on July 1 is universally celebrated. Almost every community organizes some kind of celebration during the summer months so it's worthwhile inquiring locally during your visit.

January/February
Niagara Icewine Celebrations, Niagara Peninsula *WinterCity*, Toronto
Québec Winter Carnival (➤ 60), Québec City
Winterlude, Ottawa

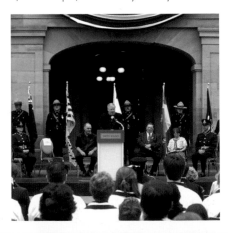

Montréal High Lights Festival, Montréal

March *SnoBreak Winter Festival,* Goose Bay, Labrador

Toronto Canada Blooms: Flower and Garden Show, Toronto

April *Blue Metropolis Literary Festival,* Montréal

World Stage International Theatre Festival, Toronto

May *Santé: International Wine Festival,* Toronto

Canadian Tulip Festival (► 60), Ottawa

June *Canada Dance Festival,* Ottawa

June/July *Festival 500 – Sharing the Voices* (► 60), St. John's (odd numbered years)

Nova Scotia International Tattoo, Halifax

Charlottetown Festival, Prince Edward Island

International Jazz Festival (► 60), Montréal

Montréal International Fireworks Competition, Montréal

July *Canada's Irish Festival,* Miramichi, New Brunswick

Just for Laughs Comedy Festival (► 60), Montréal

Festival d'été du Québec, Québec City

Les Grands Feux Loto Québec, Montmorency, Québec

Festival de Lanaudière, Joliette, Québec (July–August, dates vary year to year)

Divers/Cité – International Gay & Lesbian Pride Festival, Montréal (July–August, dates vary year to year)

Kingston Buskers Rendezvous, Kingston

August *Halifax International Busker Festival,* Halifax

Atlantic Seafood Festival (► 60), Moncton, New Brunswick

Fergus Scottish Festival and Highland Games, Fergus, Ontario

Festival of the Islands, Gananoque, Ontario

Canadian National Exhibition (► 60), Toronto (18 August–4 September)

Canadian Grand Masters Fiddle Championship, Nepean, Ottawa

September *Toronto International Film Festival,* Toronto

Harvest Jazz and Blues Festival, Fredericton

Niagara Wine Festival, St. Catharines, Ontario

October *Celtic Colours International Festival,* Sydney, Cape Breton, Nova Scotia

Oktoberfest (► 60), Kitchener, Ontario

November *Canadian Aboriginal Festival,* Toronto

December *Christmas Lights Across Canada* (► 60), Ottawa

Getting there

BY AIR

Toronto International Airport

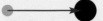

27km (17 miles) from city center

🛄 45 minutes

🚌 45 minutes

🚐 1–1.5 hours

Montréal International Airport

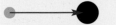

14.5km (9 miles) from city center

🚌 30 minutes

🚐 30 minutes

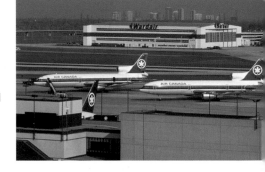

Eastern Canada's major airports are in Toronto (Toronto Lester B. Pearson International Airport; www.gtaa.com) and Montréal (Montréal-Pierre Elliott Trudeau International Airport; www.admtl.com); most visitors arrive at one or the other. There are smaller airports in Ottawa, Québec, Halifax and St. John's. The major Canadian airline is Air Canada tel: 888/247-2262 (toll free); www.aircanada.com.

Toronto's airport, Canada's largest, is 27km (17 miles) northwest of the city center. The Airport Express Bus (www.torontoairportexpress.com) to downtown hotels and the bus station runs regularly about every 30 minutes (every 20 minutes during peak times) and takes roughly 45 minutes. A cheaper option is the regular transit bus (www.ttc.ca). The Montréal-Pierre Elliott Trudeau International Airport is just 14.5km (9 miles) from downtown and L'Aérobus shuttle (www.autobus.qc.ca) runs to the bus station.

DRIVING

- Drive on the right, pass on the left.
- You can turn right at red lights, after stopping to check that the way is clear, unless otherwise signed. However, this is illegal in Montréal.
- Speed limits on highways: 100kph (60mph) or 110kph (68mph)
  Speed limits on other major roads: 70–80kph (40–50mph)
  Speed limits in urban areas and on rural routes: 50kph (30mph) or less.
- Seat belts must be worn by all people in a vehicle (drivers and passengers) in both the front and back seats and child safety seats are a legal requirement.
- Random breath-testing. Never drive under the influence of alcohol.
- Gasoline is heavily taxed. Gas stations stay open until 9–10pm (some all night). Away from the much-traveled south, gas stations may be far apart and close at 8pm.
- If you intend to drive long distances in remote areas, take out membership in the Canadian Automobile Association (www.caa.ca; South Central Ontario tel: 800/268-3750, www.caasco.on.ca; North and East Ontario tel:1-800/267-8713, www.caaneo.com; Niagara tel: 905/984-8585, www.caaniagara.net; Québec tel:1-800/686-9243, www.caaquebec.com; Maritimes tel:1-800/561-8807, www.caa.maritimes.ca). They or their local affiliate can help in case of breaking down.
- If you are a member of AAA, you are entitled to full service with the CAA if you have your membership card with you.

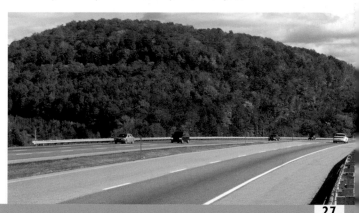

Getting around

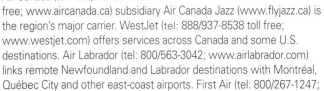

PUBLIC TRANSPORTATION
Internal flights

Air Canada (tel: 888/247-2262 toll
free; www.aircanada.ca) subsidiary Air Canada Jazz (www.flyjazz.ca) is
the region's major carrier. WestJet (tel: 888/937-8538 toll free;
www.westjet.com) offers services across Canada and some U.S.
destinations. Air Labrador (tel: 800/563-3042; www.airlabrador.com)
links remote Newfoundland and Labrador destinations with Montréal,
Québec City and other east-coast airports. First Air (tel: 800/267-1247;
www.firstair.ca) provides links from Ottawa or Montréal
with the far north.

Trains

VIA Rail (tel: 888/842-7245 toll free; www.viarail.ca)
provides most rail passenger services in Eastern
Canada. There are excellent daily services between
Montréal and Toronto, Montréal and Québec, and Montréal
and Ottawa. Trains run several times a week between Montréal and
Gaspé, and Montréal and Halifax.

Buses
Long-distance buses This is the
least expensive option and gives
access to most of the region.
Greyhound Canada (tel: 800/661-
8747 toll free; www.greyhound.ca)
serves Ontario, Québec, New
Brunswick and Nova Scotia with
cross-border links to U.S. cities.

Ferries In Nova Scotia, services link
Yarmouth with the state of Maine,
Digby with Saint John, New
Brunswick, and Caribou with Wood

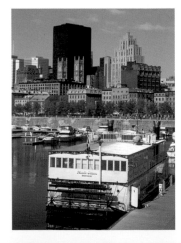

Islands, Prince Edward Island. The Nova Scotia Tourist Office can supply details. Newfoundland is linked to North Sydney, Nova Scotia, by two different ferries run by Marine Atlantic (www.marine-atlantic.ca).

Urban transportation Toronto and Montréal have excellent subway systems. The Toronto Transit System (TTC tel: 416/393-4636; www.ttc.ca), operates buses, streetcars, the subway and a light rapid transit system (LTR). The Société de Transport de Montréal (STM tel: 514/786-4636; www.stm.info), runs the métro and bus service.

TAXIS

Taxis are the most expensive option. Fares mount quickly, especially in rush-hour traffic. Cabs can be found in stands beside major hotels, at airports and at train and bus stations or can be hailed on the street or called by telephone.

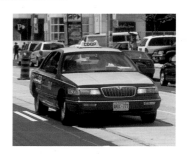

CAR RENTAL

All the major car-rental companies are represented in Eastern Canada (Avis, Budget, Dollar, Hertz, National, and Thrifty). You must be over 21, and produce identification and a valid driver's license (which you have held for at least a year).

FARES AND TICKETS

Tickets for flights, train and buses can be bought online as well as at airports, stations and ticket agents. Long-distance bus and train companies also offer passes covering various periods of unlimited travel. In Toronto, free transfers are available for continuing your journey by bus or streetcar, but must be obtained when paying the subway fare. Bus fares can be paid in cash to the driver, but you need the exact fare.

Reduced rates are available for children, students and seniors (proof of age or status required). Most museums, galleries and tourist attractions offer concessions and there are often combined ticket deals covering more than one attraction in a town or city.

Being there

TOURIST OFFICES

● **Tourism New Brunswick**

✉ P.O. Box 12345, Campbellton, New Brunswick, E3N 3T6

☎ 800/561-0123 (toll free); www.tourismnewbrunswick.ca

● **Newfoundland and Labrador Department of Tourism**

✉ P.O. Box 8700, St. John's, Newfoundland and Labrador, A1B 4J6 ☎ 800/563-6353 (toll free); www.newfoundland labrador.com

● **Nova Scotia Tourism**

✉ P.O. Box 456, Halifax, Nova Scotia, B3J 2R5 ☎ 800/565-0000 (toll free); www.novascotia.com

● **Ontario Travel**

✉ 10th Floor, Hearst Block, 900 Bay Street, Toronto, Ontario, M7A 2E1 ☎ 800/668-2746 (toll free); www.ontariotravel.net

● **Prince Edward Island Department of Tourism**

✉ P.O. Box 940, Charlottetown, Prince Edward Island, C1A 7M5

☎ 800/463-4734 (toll free); www.gov.pe.ca/visitorsguide

● **Tourisme Québec**

✉ P.O. Box 979, Montréal, Québec, H3C 2W3 ☎ 877/266-5687 (toll free); www.bonjourquebec.com

MONEY

Eastern Canada's currency is the Canadian dollar (1 dollar = 100 cents). There are $5, $10, $20, $50 and $100 bills (notorious for forgeries and can be difficult to use). Coins come as pennies (1 cent), nickels (5 cents), dimes (10 cents), quarters (25 cents), loonies ($1, so called because of the bird on them), and twonies ($2). U.S. dollars are widely accepted, but stores, restaurants, etc. might not offer the best exchange rate.

TIPS/GRATUITIES

Yes ✓ No ✗		
Restaurants (if service not included)	✓	10–15%
Cafés	✓	10%
Taxis	✓	10–15%
Porters	✓	$1–$2/bag
Chambermaids	✓	$2–$5/week
Washrooms/restrooms	✗	
Tour guides	✓	$1

POSTAL AND INTERNET SERVICES

Mail boxes are generally red, with the words "Canada Post" or "Postes Canada" written on them. For hours of post offices, ➤ 32. For more information visit www.canadapost.ca.

In all major towns and cities, internet access is available at libraries and internet cafés. There are WiFi hotspots in Montréal, Halifax, Ottawa, Toronto, and several other towns and cities in Ontario. Many hotels offer internet access, sometimes free but usually for a charge.

TELEPHONES

Outdoor public telephones are located in glass and metal booths. To make a call, lift the handset, insert the correct coin (25¢ or $1), a telephone credit card or a prepaid calling card, probably the most convenient means to make a long-distance call (available from post offices, convenience stores and newsagents), then dial.

In Toronto and Montréal include the area code, even when dialling from within the city. The toll-free numbers listed in this guide are free only when calling from within North America.

Emergency telephone numbers
Police, Fire, Ambulance: 911
(except in Prince Edward Island and Nova Scotia where you dial 0 for the operator).

International dialling codes
From Canada to:
U.S.A. 1
U.K. 011 44
France 011 33

EMBASSIES AND CONSULATES

U.S.A. ☎ 613/688-5335;
www.usembassy.gov
U.K. ☎ 613/237-1530;
http://ukincanada.fco.gov.uk/en/
Australia ☎ 613/236-0841;
www.ahc-ottawa.org

France ☎ 613/789-1795;
www.ambafrance-ca.org
Germany ☎ 613/232-1101;
www.ottawa.diplo.de

ELECTRICITY

The voltage across Eastern Canada is 110 volts, the same as in the U.S.A. Sockets require plugs with two (or three) flat prongs. Visitors from outside North America will require an adapter as well as a voltage converter.

HEALTH AND SAFETY

Sun advice In Ontario and Québec temperatures can reach the 30s °C (80s and 90s °F) so use sunscreen. Winter sun reflected off snow can cause serious sunburn so use sunscreen during outdoor activities.

Prescription drugs Over-the-counter drugs are readily available in pharmacies but out-of-province prescriptions are never accepted. If you run out of medication get a new prescription from a local doctor.

Safe water Tap water is perfectly safe to drink. When camping, boil drinking water to protect yourself against "beaver fever."

Pretty crime Although crime rates are low in Eastern Canada you should still take precautions:

● Don't leave bags or other valuables visible in your car.
● Don't wear expensive jewelry or carry large sums of money.
● In the major cities consider carrying your passport and credit cards in a pouch or belt.
● Keep to well-lit streets at night.

The Royal Canadian Mounted Police (RCMP; www.rcmp-grc.gc.ca) is the federal police force. When on duty they look like any other police force and drive cars – the famous uniform and horses are used for ceremonies.

OPENING HOURS

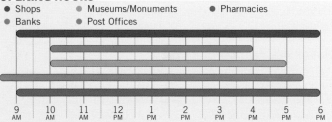

● Shops   ● Museums/Monuments   ● Pharmacies
● Banks   ● Post Offices

| 9 AM | 10 AM | 11 AM | 12 PM | 1 PM | 2 PM | 3 PM | 4 PM | 5 PM | 6 PM |

Most stores open Mon–Wed 9–6, Thu–Fri 9–9, Sat 9–5, Sun noon–5 although supermarkets and shopping malls often have longer hours.
Banks open Mon–Fri 9:30–4 but some close at 5pm or 6pm on Thu or Fri.
Post offices are open Mon–Fri 8:30–5:30 (sometimes later) and Sat am.
Museums open Tue–Sun 10–5 with art museums often opening at 11.
Most are closed Mon and some stay open until 9 one evening a week.

LANGUAGE

The official language of the province of Québec is French and New Brunswick is officially bilingual. Most Québec sights in the book are listed by their French name, followed by the English translation. For a few sights the English name is given first when this is in common use.

hello	*bonjour*	please	*s'il vous plaît*
good evening	*bonsoir*	Excuse me	*Excusez-moi*
good night	*bon nuit*	How much?	*Combien?*
goodbye	*au revoir*	open/closed	*ouvert/fermé*
yes/no	*oui/non*	Where is..?	*Où est..?*
thank you	*merci*	morning/afternoon	*matin/après-midi*
you're welcome	*bienvenue*	evening/night	*soir/nuit*
hotel/inn	*hôtel/auberge*	double room	*occupation double*
bed-and-breakfast	*gîte touristique*	one night	*une nuit*
single room	*occupation simple*	room service	*service à la chambre*
bank	*banque*	banknote	*billet de banque*
exchange office	*bureau de change*	check	*chèque*
post office	*bureau de poste*	traveler's check	*chèque de voyage*
coin	*pièce de monnaie*	credit card	*carte de credit*
restaurant	*restaurant*	menu	*menu/table d'hôte*
café	*café*	waiter	*serveur*
pub/bar	*brasserie/bar*	The check, please	*L'addition s'il vous plaît*
breakfast/lunch/ dinner	*déjeuner/dîner/ souper*	washrooms/ restrooms	*toilettes*
table	*table*		
airport/airplane	*aéroport/avion*	subway/bus/taxi	*métro/autobus/taxi*
ferry/port	*traversier/port*	station/train/tickets	*gare/train/billets*
customs/ international border	*douanes/ frontière*	entrance/exit	*entrée/sortie*
		right/left	*droite/gauche*
		straight ahead	*tout droit*
expressway/ road/street	*autoroute/ chemin/rue*	north/south/ east/west	*nord/sud/ est/ouest*

Best places to see

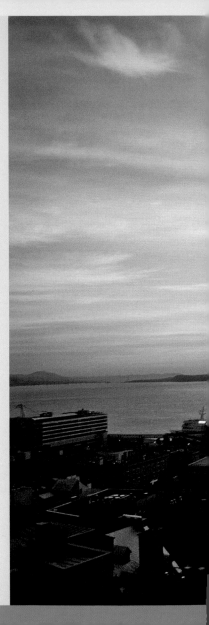

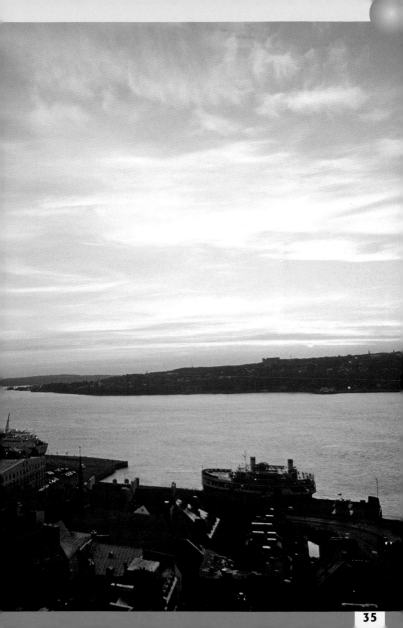

1 Canadian Museum of Civilization, Gatineau

www.civilization.ca

Their curved lines evoking the birth of the North American continent, the buildings of the Canadian Museum of Civilization are stunning, quite the most interesting architectural ensemble in Canada.

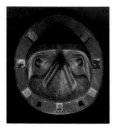

The Canadian Museum of Civilization occupies a fine site across the Ottawa River from the Canadian Parliament Buildings (➤ 156). The masterpiece of architect Douglas Cardinal, opened in 1989, the buildings suggest the emergence of man on a continent sculpted and eroded by nature. Even the Manitoba limestone cladding is significant, with its fossils dating back from early geological times. The less dramatic structure is the curatorial block. The museum proper is characterized by large glass walls and huge copper vaults and domes.

The Great Hall forms the museum's architectural centerpiece, occupying a whopping 1,782sq m (19,182sq ft) of space and with floor-to-ceiling windows rising 112m (365ft). It houses six complete log houses of the Pacific coast peoples set along a shoreline, and includes a magnificent collection of totem poles. A large contemporary sculpture by Bill Reid hangs at the far end. Called *Spirit of Haida Gwaii*, this original plaster shows a Haida canoe full of people paddling vigorously.

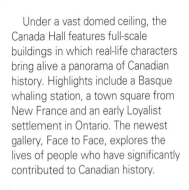

Under a vast domed ceiling, the Canada Hall features full-scale buildings in which real-life characters bring alive a panorama of Canadian history. Highlights include a Basque whaling station, a town square from New France and an early Loyalist settlement in Ontario. The newest gallery, Face to Face, explores the lives of people who have significantly contributed to Canadian history.

✚ 8D ✉ 100 Laurier Street, P.O. Box 3100, Station B, Gatineau, Québec, KIA 0M8. The museum is easily accessible from Ottawa (Ontario) by bridge ☎ 819/776-7000; 800/555-5621 (toll free) 🕐 Daily (closed Mon mid-Oct to Apr) 🖐 Expensive; free Thu 4–9. Parking charge 🍴 Restaurant ($$$), cafeteria ($), café ($) ❓ Guided tours. Craft boutique, IMAX movie theater, Children's Museum, Postal Musuem

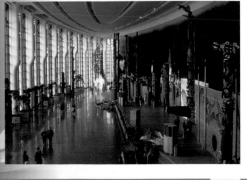

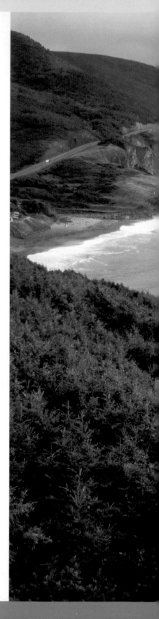

2 Cape Breton Highlands National Park

Stunning scenery of forest-clad mountains plunging down to a rocky coastline dotted with delightful bays and beaches makes this one of the most beautiful national parks in Canada.

On the northernmost tip of Nova Scotia, Cape Breton frequently features prominently on lists of the most beautiful islands in the world. The area that is preserved as the national park stretches from coast to coast just short of its northernmost tip and consists of 950sq km (366sq miles) of densely forested, rugged wilderness.

That's not to say it is inaccessible. Scenic Highway 19 – better known as the Cabot Trail (▶ 16, 70) – forms a convenient horseshoe along the coastlines and across the top of the park, with regular pull-offs for safe parking and access to the 25 trails that lead into the interior or down to secluded coves. These range from short but fascinating "leg-stretchers" to the challenging Fishing Cove hike of

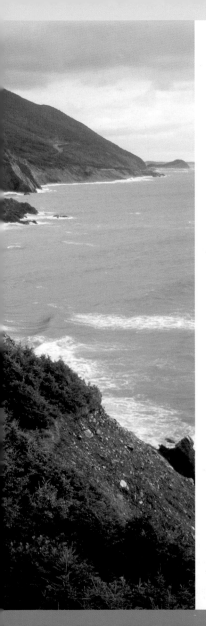

more than 15km (10 miles) from the top of MacKenzie Mountain to sea level and back. All are designed to explore this complex environment, which encompasses southern and arctic plants, and woodland that provides spectacular fall colors. The forests are home to some 40 species of mammals, including moose, coyote and lynx, and the offshore marine environment has whales, seals and a variety of seabirds. Whale-watching trips operate from Chéticamp, Pleasant Bay and Ingonish.

Check the weather before a visit – sea mists often roll in and mar the view – and try to make a first call at the excellent park center just north of Chéticamp, where there is an audio-visual program, hands-on exhibits, kids' activities, maps and information.

✚ 21J ✉ Parks Canada, Ingonish Beach, Nova Scotia B0C 1L0 ☎ 902/224-2306; www.pc.gc.ca/pnnp/ns/cbreton/ ☯ Park: daily; information center: mid-May to mid-Oct daily 9–5 (8–8 in summer) 🖐 Moderate (visitors need to buy a permit)
🍴 Restaurants and cafés at Chéticamp, Pleasant Bay and Ingonish ($–$$)
Chéticamp Information Centre
✉ Highway 19, north of Chéticamp
☎ 902/224-2306 ☯ Mid-May to mid-Oct daily 9–5 (8–8 in summer)

3 CN Tower, Toronto

www.cntower.ca

The ultimate symbol of modern Toronto, this needle-thin mast with a bulge two-thirds of the way up was the world's tallest building until a Dubai hotel eclipsed it in 2007. The view from it is nothing short of spectacular.

The CN Tower rises an incredible 553.33m (1,815ft 5in). Love it or hate it, there's no denying that it has enhanced Toronto's skyline ever since its construction in the 1970s. Glass-fronted elevators climb to the Look Out, two-thirds of the way up

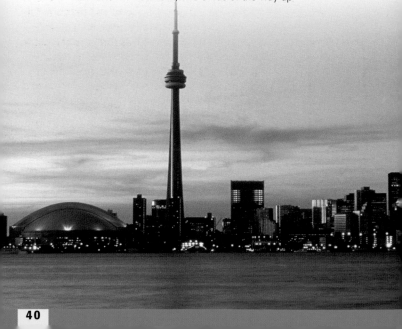

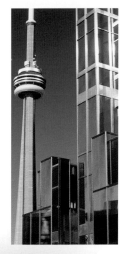

(346m, or 1,136ft, above the ground) at a stomach-churning speed of 6m (20ft) a second. The city's landmarks can easily be identified either from inside or from an outdoor observatory one floor down. Those with a good head for heights can even look directly down at the ground while standing on a glass floor.

Don't miss the ascent to the SkyPod, another 33 floors up, or 447m (1,465ft) above the ground. This is the world's highest man-made observatory and the view is superb. Visibility can exceed 160km (100 miles) and, with luck, you will be able to make out the spray of Niagara Falls and the city of Rochester, New York state, across Lake Ontario. You should be aware, however, that the tower can sway up to 1.8m (6ft) from the vertical on windy days – a normal but somewhat unnerving sensation.

The CN Tower was not primarily intended as a tourist attraction, but a telecommunications tower. During the 1960s, Toronto experienced a construction boom that transformed the skyline from one characterized by relatively low buildings, into one dotted with skyscrapers. These new buildings caused serious communications problems as they got in the way of the airwaves. However, the CN Tower, with microwave receptors at 338m (1,109ft) and topped by an antenna, effectively solved these difficulties.

✚ *Toronto 2b* ✉ 301 Front Street, Toronto, Ontario, M5V 2T6 ☎ 416/868-6937 ⏱ Daily; closed Dec 25; hours of operation adjusted seasonally ✋ Expensive ⑪ 360 Restaurant ($$$), cafés ($) Ⓤ Union Station ❓ Souvenir shops. Long lines during peak times and seasons

4 Mont-Royal, Montréal

www.lemontroyal.qc.ca

Mont-Royal Park, the jewel in Montréal's crown, was created by the landscape architect Frederick Law Olmstead, and offers magnificent views of the city and river from its Chalet viewpoint.

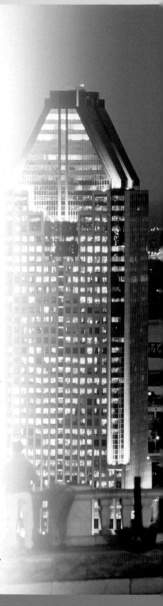

At the center of the island of Montréal and deep in the heart of the city, the bulky lump of Mont-Royal rises 228m (750ft). "La Montagne" (the Mountain) is not only a lovely park, but it is also part of the city's soul. It provides a wonderful oasis of greenery in the center of the bustling metropolis, and as such is popular with residents year-round.

In 1876, the city expropriated the land at the top of the mountain for a hefty $1 million, and then invited Frederick Law Olmstead (famous for designing Central Park in New York) to landscape it. Near the summit, the large stone Smith House, built in 1858, acts as a visitors' centre, with an exhibition about the park and a café.

High above the bustle of the city, the Chalet offers views that are nothing less than spectacular. The downtown highrises are particularly prominent. The mighty St. Lawrence can be seen winding its way around the city, and on clear days the Adirondack Mountains of northern New York state are visible, as are the Green Mountains of Vermont. The view is equally spectacular at night.

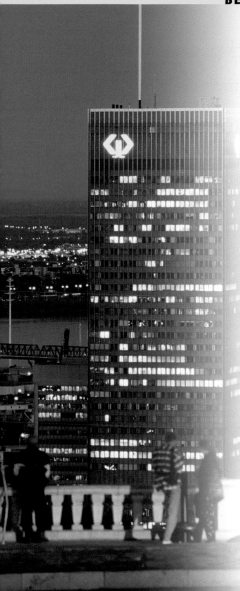

The wide, flat St. Lawrence valley is punctuated by a series of small, rather dramatic peaks like Mont-Royal, which were created about 60 million years ago during a period of tectonic activity. These igneous plugs are known as the Collines Montérégiennes (Monteregian Hills), from *mons regius*, the Latin name for Mont-Royal. According to most historians, the city's name also derives from Mont-Royal.

✚ *Montréal 1e (off map)*
✉ Parc du Mont-Royal, Voie Camillien-Houde, Montréal, Québec ☎ 514/843-8240
🕐 Daily 🎟 Free; parking charge 🍽 Cafeteria ($) at Smith House 🚌 11 from Mont-Royal métro station and rue Côte-des-Nieges ❓ Accessible on foot from avenue du Parc, avenue des Pins, and rue Côte-des-Nieges via Trafalgar staircase (200 steps; allow 20 mins)

5 Niagara Falls

www.niagaraparks.com

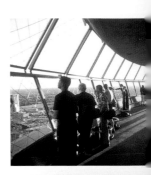

In 1678, French explorer Louis Hennepin exclaimed, "The universe does not afford its parallel," a sentiment still echoed by the millions of people who flock to Niagara Falls every year.

This famous waterfall is one of the best-known, most visited and most photographed sights in the world. Around 14 million people visit it annually, taking an estimated 100 million photographs. The fascination of watching all that "thundering water" (the meaning of the First Nations word Niagara) endlessly flowing over the rock edge has a totally mesmerizing effect. Few are disappointed; many are more impressed than they expected to be. Niagara Falls are quite simply fantastic.

Just before it reaches tiny Goat Island, the Niagara River divides into two. About 10 percent of the water heads for the American Falls (so called because they are on the U.S. side of the river), which are more than 300m (985ft) wide and 54m (176ft) high. The rest of the water heads for the Canadian, or Horseshoe Falls, which are named for their shape and are nearly 800m (2,625ft) wide and about 51m (167ft) high. The water crashes over the falls at the incredible rate of 155 million liters (40 million gallons) per minute.

At Table Rock, you can approach the very edge of the Horseshoe Falls, the point where the tumultuous water plunges over the cliff. It is incredibly impressive, but it can also be wet on windy days. From here you can descend by elevator

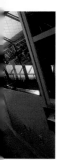

to two outdoor observation decks directly behind the falls – also impressive and wet. And nobody should miss the exciting (and wet) *Maid of the Mist* boat trip.

🚩 8B ✉ Niagara Parks Commission ☎ 905/371-0254; 877/642-7275 ✋ Parking: expensive. Boat tour: expensive 🍴 Elements on the Falls Restaurant ($$$), cafés ($) 🚌 People Mover bus: daily, Mar–Dec 🚢 *Maid of the Mist*: daily, late Apr or early May–late Oct; Niagara Parkway (➤ 173) ❓ Welcome Centers are located at Table Rock, *Maid of the Mist* ticket booth and various locations

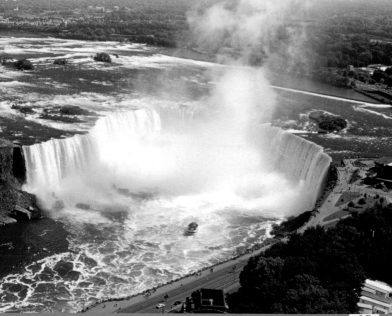

6 Rocher Percé, Gaspésie

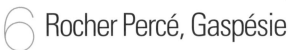

www.rocherperce.com

A massive pierced limestone rock sits seemingly at anchor just off the tiny community of Percé at the end of the magnificent Gaspé Peninsula.

Rocher Percé is a limestone block formed from layers of sediment deposited on the seabed about 375 million years ago. It soars high above the surrounding sand to 88m (289ft) and is an amazing 438m (1,437ft) in length. At its eastern end, it is pierced by an arch. Once there were two arches here, but in 1848, during a storm, one collapsed to leave the separate pinnacle now known as the Obelisk.

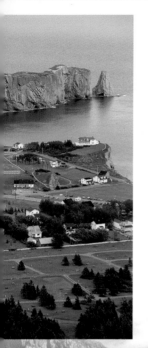

Renowned for the beauty of its site, the village of Percé is blessed with a varied topography, and nowhere else on the peninsula are the geological forces that shaped Gaspésie more evident. Yellowish limestone and red conglomerate rock have been squeezed, folded and manipulated into an incredible variety of protruding cliffs, deep bays and craggy hills.

You can park in the town and walk out to Rocher Percé – or even around it if the tide is out. Every cape and headland in the community offers a different view. Mont-Ste.-Anne, the craggy peak dominating the town, has particularly splendid panoramas, although the path leading up it is steep (the trail begins beside the church; allow 1.5 hours to reach the summit). You get another wonderful view of Rocher Percé by taking the boat tour to Bonaventure Island, which passes close to the rock before making a circular tour of the island famous for its seabirds, notably its huge gannet colony.

✚ 20J 🍽 Variety of restaurants and cafés in Percé ❷ Boat tours in summer only (details available from tourist information office) ℹ Information touristique de Percé: 142 Route 132, Percé, Québec, G0C 2L0 ☎ 418/782-5448

7

Science North, Sudbury

www.sciencenorth.on.ca

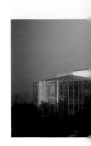

Set in an oval crater in the Precambrian Canadian Shield, Sudbury is home to a stunning science center hewn out of the rock below two glittering snowflake-shaped buildings.

Even if you find science the most boring thing on Earth, you will be impressed by Science North, in Sudbury, deep in northern Ontario's mining belt. The two unusual snowflake buildings, representing the glaciation that sculpted the Canadian landscape, are clad with stainless steel, the main ingredient of which is locally mined nickel.

An underground rock tunnel links the two buildings, ending in a huge underground cavern representing the crater in which the center sits. From the cavern, visitors proceed to the exhibit floors along a glass-enclosed ramp that offers views of Ramsey Lake and part of a fault that runs through the rock at this point. This rock fault was deliberately excavated for its geological interest.

As far as the exhibits are concerned, you have to roll up your sleeves and get involved. You can have a go at building a robot in the LEGO Mindstorms Robotics Lab, and if that doesn't appeal, you can hold a snake or watch beavers in action. WaterWorks: Soak Up the Science! is a new exhibit all about H2O, from making a rainbow to learning about water power through interactive games. There are also laser shows and IMAX

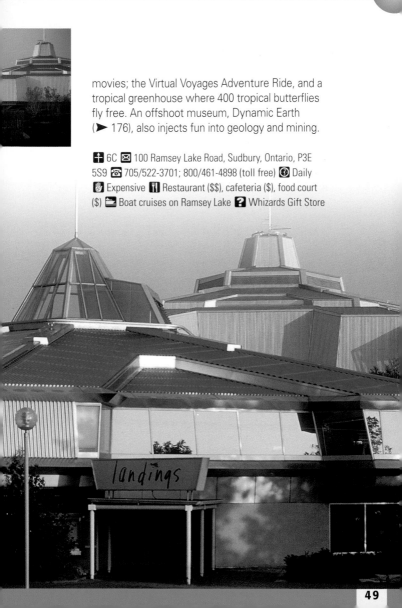

movies; the Virtual Voyages Adventure Ride, and a tropical greenhouse where 400 tropical butterflies fly free. An offshoot museum, Dynamic Earth (➤ 176), also injects fun into geology and mining.

🕇 6C ✉ 100 Ramsey Lake Road, Sudbury, Ontario, P3E 5S9 ☎ 705/522-3701; 800/461-4898 (toll free) 🕓 Daily 🖐 Expensive 🍴 Restaurant ($$), cafeteria ($), food court ($) 🚢 Boat cruises on Ramsey Lake ❓ Whizards Gift Store

8 Signal Hill, St. John's

www.pc.gc.ca

The Newfoundland capital has a spectacular site on the slopes of a natural harbor whose narrow entrance is guarded by the great rock of Signal Hill.

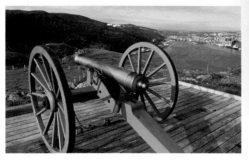

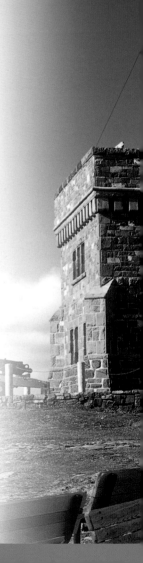

No visit to St. John's would be complete without a climb up Signal Hill for panoramic views of the city, harbor and coastline. A calm day is best for the excursion – if there is even a light breeze in the city, the wind will be strong on Signal Hill. The cliffs rise sharply to form this rocky outcrop facing the Atlantic Ocean. At the top stands Cabot Tower, the city's best-known landmark, built in 1897 to commemorate the 400th anniversary of John Cabot's visit to Newfoundland. From here, you can look straight down into The Narrows, the 200m wide (650ft) entrance to the harbor, while to the southeast is Cape Spear, North America's most easterly point.

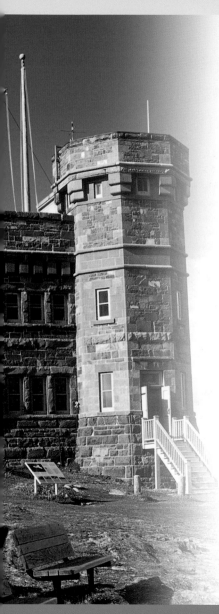

As its name suggests, Signal Hill has long been used for signalling. From the early 18th century, flags were flown from its summit to alert local merchants to the approach of their vessels. In 1901, a different type of communication took place when Guglielmo Marconi received the first transatlantic wireless signal from Poldhu in Cornwall, England. That letter "s" in Morse code traversed more than 2,700km (1,700 miles) to make history.

Today a national historic park, Signal Hill has a visitor center and a great trail system. From Cabot Tower, you can walk over to Queen's Battery or to Ladies Lookout at 160m (525ft). Avid hikers can descend the North Head to The Narrows via a steep trail on the ocean side.

✚ 23L ✉ Signal Hill Road, St. John's, Newfoundland and Labrador, A1C 5M9 ☎ 709/772-5367 🕐 Daily. Visitor center: mid-May to mid-Oct daily 8:30–8; mid-Oct to mid-May Mon–Fri 8:30–4:30 🖐 Signal Hill: free. Visitor center: inexpensive 🍴 Picnic facilities ❓ Military drills are performed by cadets Jul–Aug. Gift shop in Cabot Tower

9 Terrasse Dufferin and Promenade des Gouverneurs, Québec City

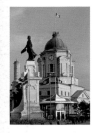

Admiring the city from the Dufferin Terrace and then following the spectacular Governors' Walk as it clings to the cliff face is one of the glories of a visit to Québec.

The Terrasse Dufferin (Dufferin Terrace) is a wide wooden boardwalk suspended high above the St. Lawrence River, offering magnificent views over the surrounding country. Extending for a total of 670m (2,200ft), it is popular year-round, day and night. On summer evenings, there are street performers, while in the winter, you can try the toboggan slide.

The history of Terrasse Dufferin starts in 1620 with Samuel de Champlain, whose statue stands in front of the Château Frontenac. He constructed the Château St. Louis here, which served as the residence of first the French, and later the British governors until it was destroyed by fire in 1834. At that time, the British governor, Lord Durham, built a platform over the ruins and allowed public access. The structure was then extended on a couple of occasions, notably in 1879 by Governor General Lord Dufferin, whose name it commemorates.

From the terrace's southern end, and accessed by a steep flight of stairs, a spectacular boardwalk

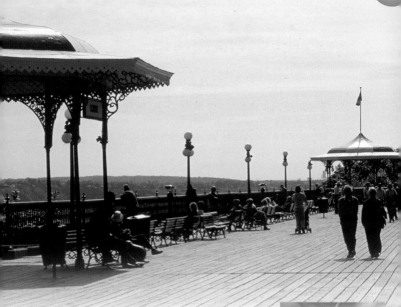

inaugurated in 1960 clings to the cliff about 90m (300ft) above the river. This is the Promenade des Gouverneurs (Governors' Walk), which goes around the outer walls of the Citadelle (➤ 127) with splendid views of the St. Lawrence, the Basse-Ville (Lower Town), Île d'Orléans and the opposite shore of the river as far as the mountains of northern Maine on a clear day. If you don't mind climbing its 310 steps, it provides an excellent means of getting to the Plains of Abraham, site of the decisive battle in the Seven Years' War.

✚ 10E ③ Terrasse Dufferin: daily. Promenade des Gouverneurs: May–Oct daily ✋ Free 🍴 Restaurants and cafés nearby ❓ Terrasse Dufferin adjoins place d'Armes in front of Château Frontenac. Promenade des Gouverneurs runs from the southern end of Terrasse Dufferin to avenue du Cap-Diamant in National Battlefields Park

10 Whale-watching, Tadoussac

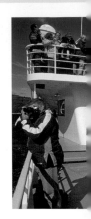

The rich waters at the point where the Saguenay River joins the St. Lawrence have long attracted giant mammals of the deep, and have made Tadoussac a famous whale-watching center.

Every day, the salty tides of the St. Lawrence River sweep into the mouth of the Saguenay, and in its turn the main stream is invaded by the fresh waters of its tributary. This mixture of waters has created a rich ecosystem where plankton flourishes, and that draws in small creatures such as krill, shrimp and

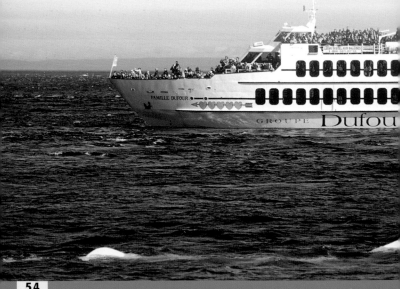

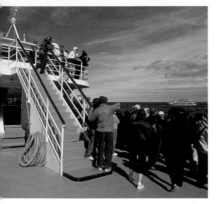

capelin which, in their turn, attract larger predators. A resident population of about 500 beluga, or white whales, haunts these waters. Fin and minke whales are also frequently viewed off Tadoussac, and occasionally humpback whales are sighted.

Tadoussac has a fine site on the cliffs and sand dunes along the north shore of the St. Lawrence, but it is rare to spot whales from the shore. The St. Lawrence is more than 10km (6 miles) wide at this point, and it is mid-river, miles from shore, where the whales frolic, great jets of water issuing from their blowholes just before they surface.

In the summer, a procession of small boats leaves Tadoussac wharf, offering a variety of tours. The views of the town and the mouth of the Saguenay are magnificent. Standing on a shoal close to the intersection of these two important waterways is the Prince Light, a 15m-high (50ft) lighthouse that was constructed after the Prince of Wales' ship ran aground here in the 1880s.

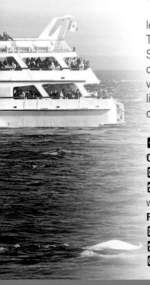

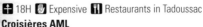

✚ 18H ♿ Expensive 🍴 Restaurants in Tadoussac

Croisières AML

✉ 124 rue St-Pierre, Québec City, Québec, G1K 4A7

☎ 418/692-2634; 800/563-4643 (toll free);
www.croisieresaml.com 🕐 May–Oct daily

Famille Dufour Croisières

✉ 22 quai St.-André, Québec City, Québec, G1K 9B7

☎ 418/692-0222; 800/463-5250 (toll free); www.dufour.ca

🕐 May–Oct daily

Best things to do

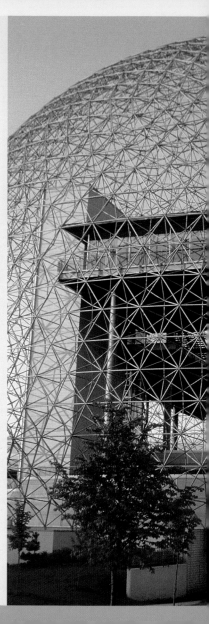

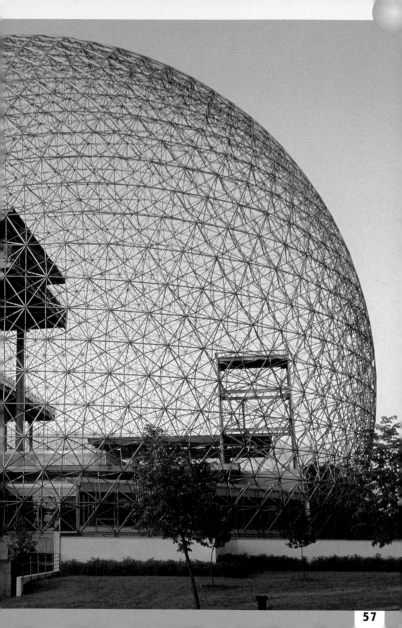

Good places to have lunch

Auberge Baker ($$$)

Traditional Québec food in an old French house between Québec City and Ste-Anne-de-Beaupré. Guests are seated either in the original section, dating from 1840, or a new, more airy addition. The menu offers both traditional and "contemporary" dishes.

✉ 8790 chemin Royale, Château-Richer, Québec ☎ 418/824-4478

Le Café du Château ($)

Great salads and light lunches in the Governor's Garden, Château Ramezay Museum, Old Montréal.

✉ 280 rue Notre-Dame Est, Montréal, Québec ☎ 514/861-1112
🕐 May–Sep only

Café l'Entrée ($)

Spectacular location in the Great Hall of the National Gallery of Canada; the menu emphasizes delicious, simply prepared foods.

✉ 380 Sussex Drive, Ottawa, Ontario ☎ 613/991-4060

Café-Restaurant du Musée ($$)

Excellent café in the Musée du Québec serving all-Québec produce; outdoor terrace in summer.

✉ Parc des Champs-de-Bataille, Québec City, Québec ☎ 418/644-6780

Cheapside Café ($)

Elegant café in the Art Gallery of Nova Scotia offering excellent light lunches and the chance to meet local politicians – the Legislature is across the street.

✉ 1723 Hollis Street, Halifax, Nova Scotia ☎ 902/424-7542

Chocolaterie and Patisserie Fackelman/The Schnitzel Parlor ($)

Beside the St. John River just west of the city, this cosy place serves hearty German food and irresistible desserts. Reservations are required.

✉ 2785 Woodstock Road, Fredericton, New Brunswick ☎ 506/450-2520

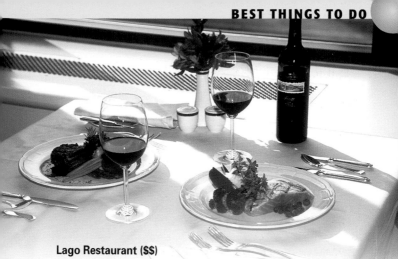

Lago Restaurant ($$)

Stylish place in Queen's Quay Terminal (▶ 72) with great food and wonderful views of the lake. Dine on the big lakeside patio or in the chic interior.

✉ 207 Queen's Quay West, Queen's Quay Terminal, Toronto, Ontario
☎ 416/848-0005

Lake House Restaurant ($$)

Simple, charming restaurant in Science North, overlooking Ramsey Lake. The menu is extensive and ranges from simple salads and sandwiches to filet mignon.

✉ 100 Ramsey Lake Road, Sudbury, Ontario ☎ 705/522-3701, ext. 505

Mavor's Bistro ($$)

Pleasant café with a long menu of bistro-style fare in the Confederation Centre of the Arts.

✉ 145 Richmond Street, Charlottetown, Prince Edward Island
☎ 902/628-6107

Restaurant Acadien ($)

Charming restaurant in the museum and craft shop serving Acadian specialties including meat pies and chowder, served by staff in traditional dress; on the Cabot Trail.

✉ 744 Main Street, Chéticamp, Cape Breton, Nova Scotia ☎ 902/224-3207

Annual events

Winter Carnival, Québec City: Parade, ice sculptures and canoe races across the ice-strewn St. Lawrence (Jan–Feb).

Canadian Tulip Festival, Ottawa: A rite of spring; more than 3 million tulips decorate the city (May).

Festival 500 – Sharing the Voices, St. John's, Newfoundland: International festival of choral singing, with choirs from all over the world (Jun/Jul).

International Jazz Festival, Montréal: More than 500 shows, 350 of them outdoors and free, in the heart of downtown Montréal (Jun/Jul).

Just for Laughs Comedy Festival, Montréal: 11 days of laughter, with top comedians and free outdoor shows (Jul).

Royal Nova Scotia International Tattoo, Halifax: Pipe bands, Highland dancers, and military displays for 10 days (Jul).

Atlantic Seafood Festival, Moncton, New Brunswick: Top chefs prepare some of the world's best seafood (Aug).

Canadian National Exhibition, Toronto: Huge annual exhibition of just about everything (Aug).

Oktoberfest, Kitchener, Ontario: the people of Kitchener invite everyone to sample their Bavarian-style festival of beer, dancing and all things German (Oct).

Christmas Lights Across Canada, Ottawa: Nearly 300,000 lights illuminate the capital to coincide with displays held across the country (Dec).

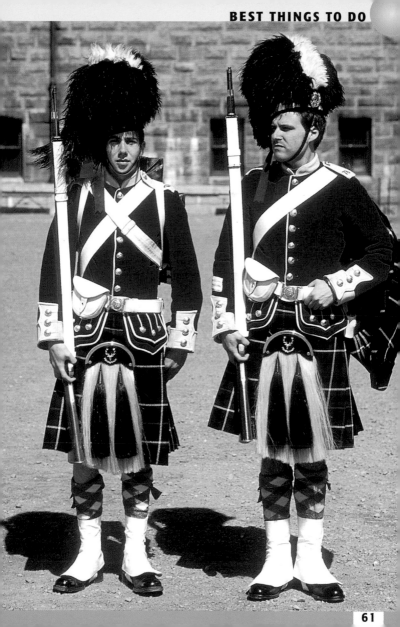

Train and boat trips

TRAIN
Agawa Canyon (Ontario)
From Sault Ste. Marie, a splendid day trip north through the wilderness of the Canadian Shield with a stop in Agawa Canyon.
☎ 800/242-9287 (toll free); 705/946-7300 (Algoma Central);
www.agawacanyontourtrain.com ⏱ Early Jun to mid-Oct

Polar Bear Express (Ontario)
From Cochrane, a 12-hour return trip north to Moosonee at Arctic tidewater on the shores of James Bay.
☎ 800/265-2356 (toll free); 705/272-5338 (Ontario Northland);
www.ontarionorthland.ca ⏱ Late Jun–late Aug

BOAT
Bonaventure Island
The island is famous for its seabirds. Boats take a circular route around the island and pass close to the Rocher Percé (➤ 46–47).

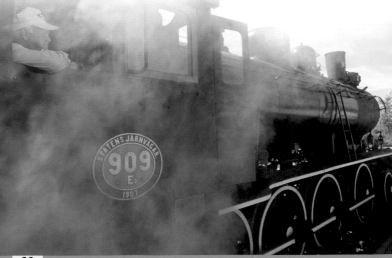

Alternatively, walk across the island for a closer view of the birds.
☎ 877/782-2974 (toll free); 418/782-2974 🕐 Mid-May to mid-Oct daily 9–5

Maid of the Mist at Niagara Falls (➤ 45)

Thousand Islands (➤ 176)
To experience the area to the fullest, you should take a boat trip.
Some trips stop to visit the amazing six-story extravaganza, Boldt
Castle, on Heart Island, built 1900–1904 by George C. Boldt.
🚢 Boat tours to Thousand Islands (expensive) run daily, May–Oct
✉ Gananoque Boat Line: 6 Water Street, Gananoque ☎ 888/717-4837 (toll
free); 613/382-2144; www.ganboatline.com ✉ Rockport Boat Line Ltd:
23 Front Street, Rockport ☎ 800/563-8687 (toll free); 613/659-3402;
www.rockportcruises.com ✉ Kingston 1000 Islands Cruises: 263 Ontario
Street, Kingston ☎ 800/848-1000; 613/549-5544; www.ktic.ca ❓ The castle
is on US soil so passports are required

Western Brook Pond
The only way to properly appreciate this lake is to walk to its
shore and take the two-hour boat trip along its length. The lake is
oligotrophic and has minimal plant life, making its waters pure.
☎ 888/458-2016 (toll free); 709/458-2016; www.bontours.ca 🕐 Jul–Aug
daily 10am, 1pm, 4pm; Jun and Sep 1pm

Whale-watching off Cape Breton
Tours by cabin cruiser or Zodiac inflatable boats (the latter can get
in closer to the whales) depart from Pleasant Bay. Pilot, minke,
humpback and fin are the most likely whales to see.
Cabot Trail Whale Watching ☎ 866/688-2424 (toll free) 🕐 Jul–Oct daily,
11, 1:30, 4 (also 6:30 in Jul)
Captain Mark's Whale and Seal Cruise ☎ 888/754-5112 (toll free);
902/224-1316 🕐 Jun 11:30, 1, 3; Jul–Oct 9:30, 11:30, 1, 3, 5

Whale-watching off Tadoussac (➤ 54–55)

Sports venues

In addition to the sports events listed, each of the stadiums below doubles as a venue for live music and large entertainment events.

HALIFAX, NOVA SCOTIA
Metro Centre
This is the home of the Halifax Mooseheads hockey team, not in the National Hockey League (NHL), but with enthusiastic fans.

✉ Brunswick Street ☎ 902/451-1221; www.halifaxmetrocentre.com

MONCTON, NEW BRUNSWICK
Moncton Coliseum
The Moncton Wildcats hockey team, not in the NHL, play the Mooseheads (see above) and teams from Québec.

✉ 377 Killam Drive ☎ 888/720-5600 (toll free); 506/857-4100; www.monctoncoliseum.com

MONTRÉAL
Bell Centre
They say that hockey is not a sport in Montréal but a religion. The Montréal Canadiens, or "Habs", have a fanatical following.

✉ 1260 rue de la Gauchetière ☎ 514/790-1245; 514/989-2841 (ticket office); www.centrebell.ca 🚇 Bonaventure, Lucien L'Allier

Olympic Stadium
Built for the 1976 Olympic Games, it's now home to the Montréal Expos, one of two Canadian teams playing major league baseball.

✉ 4549 avenue Pierre du Coubertin ☎ 514/252-4141; www.rio.gouv.qc.ca

OTTAWA
Scotiabank Place
Home to the capital's NHL team, the Ottawa Senators and also the Ottawa Rebels who play Canada's official national game: lacrosse.

✉ 1000 Palladium Drive, Kanata ☎ 613/599-0100; www.scotiabankplace.com

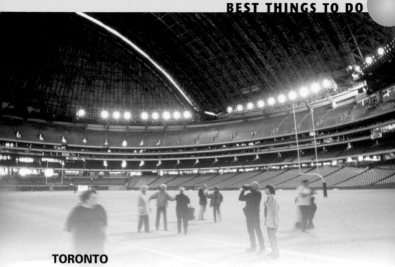

TORONTO
Air Canada Centre
Expect big crowds and excitement when Toronto Maple Leafs play hockey at home, especially if they're up against arch-rivals the Montréal Canadiens. The centre also hosts games by the Toronto Raptors NBA team and the Toronto Rock lacrosse team.

✉ 40 Bay Street ☎ 416/815-5500; www.theaircanadacentre.com
🚇 Union Station

BMO Field
Opened in 2007, this is Canada's first stadium constructed specifically for soccer, and can seat 20,000 spectators. It is the home of both Toronto FC and Canada's national soccer team.

✉ 170 Princes' Boulevard, Exhibition Place ☎ 416/263-5700; 416/360-GOAL (ticket office); www.bmofield.com 🚇 Union Station, then 509 streetcar west
🚌 GO train to Exhibition

Rogers Centre
This superb stadium is the home the Toronto Blue Jays, who have won the baseball World Series twice. It also hosts the Argonauts, who play in the Canadian Football League.

✉ 1 Blue Jays Way ☎ 416/341-1707; www.rogerscentre.com 🚇 Union Station, then via Skywalk

Places to take the children

ATLANTIC PROVINCES
CAVENDISH, PRINCE EDWARD ISLAND
Avonlea

The *Anne of Green Gables* books by Lucy Maud Montgomery were set on Prince Edward Island (➤ 100–101). Children can relive the stories, explore the farm and attend an old-fashioned school. Tea room.

✉ 8779 Route 6 ☎ 902/963-3050; www.avonlea.ca 🕓 Mid-Jun to Sep daily 🖐 Expensive

ONTARIO
CAMBRIDGE
African Lion Safari

Southwest of Toronto. Home to more than 1,000 African animals – including lions, elephants and monkeys – which roam freely in large game reserves that you can drive through.

✉ Safari Road, Rural Route 1 ☎ 800/461-9453 (toll free); 519/623-2620; www.lionsafari.com 🕓 Late Apr to mid-Oct daily 🖐 Expensive

LONDON
Children's Museum

Experience life in the Arctic, dig up dinosaur bones, hunt for cave dwellers, or dress up like an astronaut.

✉ 21 Wharncliffe Road South ☎ 519/434-5726; www.londonchildrensmuseum.ca 🕓 Tue–Sun 10–5 (Fri to 8); also Mon Jun–Aug and public hols 🖐 Inexpensive

NIAGARA FALLS
Marineland

Huge aquarium complex with beluga whales, sea lions, walruses and interactive pools with underwater viewing panels. Children can help feed the animals and there are thrill rides.

✉ 7657 Portage Road ☎ 905/356-9565; www.marineland.ca 🕓 Late May to mid-Oct daily 🚌 Niagara People Mover bus (Apr–Dec) 🖐 Expensive

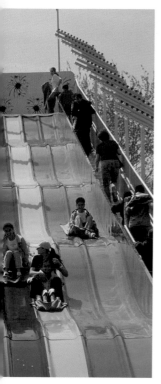

OTTAWA
Aboriginal Experiences

Aboriginal Experiences brings aboriginal culture to life with tepees, totem poles, canoes, singing, dancing and storytelling – complete with restaurant serving aboriginal food.

✉ Victoria Island ☎ 877/811-3233 (toll free); 613/564-9494; www.aboriginalexperiences.com
🕐 Late Jun–early Sep daily 💷 Moderate

QUÉBEC
MONTRÉAL
Centre des Sciences de Montréal

Engrossing science center on the waterfront in the Old Port of Montréal. Hands-on exhibits and an IMAX movie theater.

✉ quai King Edward ☎ 877/496-4724 (toll free); 514/496-4724; www.centredessciencesdemontreal.com
🕐 Daily 🚇 Place d'Armes then short walk 💷 Expensive

VAUGHAN
Paramount Canada's Wonderland

This is Canada's premier theme park containing more than 200 attractions for all ages, including North America's best selection of roller coasters, a water park, rides for small children and live shows.

✉ 9580 Jane Street, off Highway 400, Rutherford Road exit ☎ 905/832-8131; www.canadaswonderland.com 🕐 Early May and Sep–early Oct Sat–Sun from 10am; mid-May to end Aug daily from 10am, closing time varies 🚌 Wonderland Express; GO Bus from Yorkdale and York Mills subway stations in Toronto; 165A from Toronto, 4, 20 within York region 💷 Expensive

Great museums

Canada Aviation Museum (➤ 152–153)
The museum, housed in a hangar, is part of the Canada Science and Technology Corporation. This has an excellent collection of vintage aircraft through to contemporary craft.

Canada Science and Technology Museum (➤ 153)
Easily recognized by the lighthouse outside, this large, hands-on museum covers astronomy, space travel, computers and communication as well as many other scientific and technological advances. Largest of its kind in the country.

Canadian Museum of Civilization (➤ 36–37)
A wonderful museum presenting Canada's history in a lively and entertaining way. The building itself is also impressive.

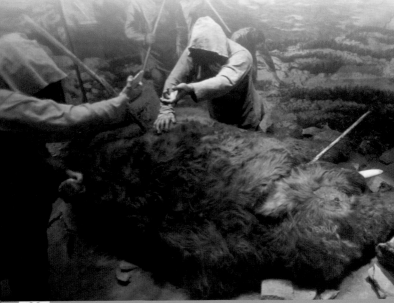

Canadian War Museum (► 154)

In 2005, the museum moved to a new location with double the original exhibition space for its interesting displays celebrating Canada's military history.

Maritime Museum of the Atlantic (► 88)

This museum presents the fascinating history of seafaring in Halifax. Life-size and model ships and a recreated chandlery are highlights.

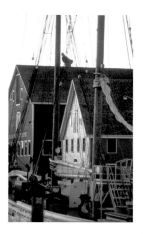

Musée d'Archéologie et d'Histoire de Montréal (► 117)

This museum devoted to archeology opened in 1992 in a strikingly modern building.

Musée d'Art Contemporain, Montréal (► 118)

The only museum in the city that specializes in contemporary art. It's part of the downtown place-des-Arts complex.

Musée des Beaux-Arts de Montréal (► 118)

Musée de la Civilisation, Québec City (► 128)

Royal Ontario Museum (► 164–165)

Canada's largest museum, and still expanding, is certain to have something that will interest all age groups. Among its more than 6 million items is a superb collection of Chinese art.

Science North (► 48–49)

Lively with lots of hands-on activities – this will appeal to children and adults alike.

Scenic drives

Acadian Coastal Drive, New Brunswick
Tracing the Atlantic coast from the Nova Scotia border to
Dalhousie, this stunning drive incorporates glorious beaches,
delightful fishing villages, the Kouchibouguac National Park and
the gorgeous Chaleur Bay.

Appalachian Range Route, New Brunswick
Weave your way through this ancient landscape of mountains,
forests, rivers and lakes that extends from the Saint John River
valley to the coast at Chaleur Bay, with the highest peak in the
Maritimes, Mount Carleton, along the way.

Bonne Bay, Newfoundland
Cutting into the Long Range Mountains within Gros Morne
National Park (➤ 95), Bonne Bay stretches deep inland from
the Gulf of St. Lawrence. Route 430, hugging the shore on the
northern side, and Route 431 along the southern side, are
equally scenic.

Cabot Trail, Nova Scotia
Breathtaking views mark this trail which encircles the Cape Breton
Highlands National Park (➤ 38–39) and its forest-cloaked
mountains and rugged coastline.

Fundy Trail, New Brunswick
Experience the highest tides in the world on a route that takes in
the Hopewell Rocks (➤ 96), the Fundy National Park (➤ 94), the
incredible Reversing Falls at Saint John and pretty St. Andrews-by-
the-Sea (➤ 101).

Georgian Bay, Ontario
Beautiful Georgian Bay, dotted with wooded islands, is an offshoot
of Lake Huron. From Wasaga Beach, on Nottawasaga Bay, take
Highway 26 west through Collingwood and Meaford, then loop

round through Annan and Leith to reach Owen Sound, from where you can drive north to the tip of the Bruce Peninsula.

Navigators' Route, Québec
This evocatively named route follows the southern shore of the St. Lawrence River, just east of Québec City, with wonderful views across to the mountains on the north shore. It passes through attractive villages redolent of seafaring heritage.

Niagara Parkway (➤ 173), Ontario
Historic sites, lush vineyards and views of the Niagara River form this route, with the breathtaking Niagara Falls (➤ 44–45) along the way. The Parkway finishes up in the charming little town of Niagara-on-the-Lake (➤ 172) on the shore of Lake Ontario.

North Cape Coastal Drive, Prince Edward Island
From Summerside, this circuit around Prince Edward Island's northwest coast visits fabulous secluded beaches and communities with rich First Nations and Acadian cultures. At low tide, you can walk from North Cape to the longest natural rock reef in North America.

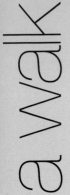

through the heart of Toronto

Start at City Hall. Cross over Bay Street, then take Albert Street and enter the Eaton Centre (➤ 79). Exit on Yonge Street and turn right. Turn left at King Street.

To your right is Scotia Plaza, across the street is Commerce Court (Canadian Imperial Bank of Commerce), ahead First Canadian Place and Toronto-Dominion Centre.

Turn left on Bay Street; cross Wellington Street.

To your right on Bay, the triangular gold-sheathed towers house the Royal Bank of Canada.

Mid-block enter Brookfield Place (left).

This elegant galleria, five floors high, incorporates two older buildings and two unusually shaped office towers.

Follow Bay Street past Union Station and under the railroad tracks. Continue under the Gardiner Expressway to the waterfront. Turn right and follow the pathway around York Street slip to Queen's Quay Terminal.

Queen's Quay Terminal houses more than 30 high-end stores, galleries and restaurants.

Follow York Street and the Teamway covered sidewalk back under the expressway and railroad. Cross Front Street and turn right at Wellington Street.

On both sides are the black-glass buildings of the Toronto-Dominion Centre.

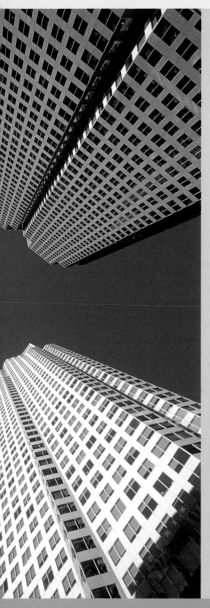

Enter the Maritime Life Tower (right), with its wonderful Inuit art. Cross Wellington Street, and walk into the courtyard of the TD Centre.

Life-size bronze cows sit chewing the cud, the work of Saskatchewan sculptor Joe Fafard.

Cross King Street and enter First Canadian Place. Descend by escalator into the PATH, a subterranean network of corridors and walkways. Follow signs back to City Hall.

Distance 4.8km (3 miles)
Time 2–2.5 hours, excluding visits
Start/end point Nathan Phillips Square, in front of Toronto City Hall, Queen Street West
✚ *Toronto 3c*
🜚 Queen, Osgoode
Lunch Pumpernickel's Deli ($$) ✉ Queens Quay Terminal ☎ 416/861-0226

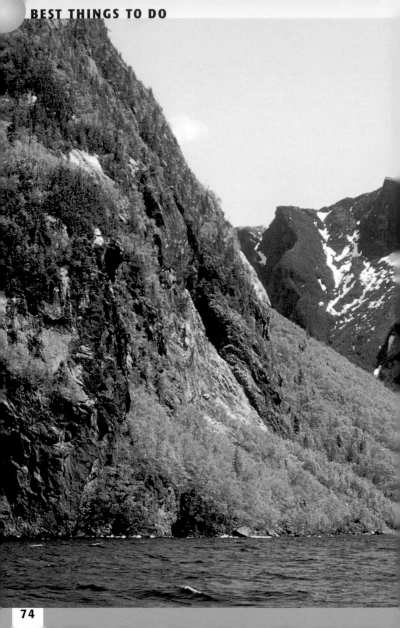

Stunning views

Cape Breton Highlands National Park (➤ 38–39)

Citadel Hill, Halifax (➤ 86)
Views across the harbor and the two bridges across The Narrows.

From the CN Tower (➤ 40–41)

Gros Morne National Park (➤ 95)
Designated a UNESCO World Heritage Site because of its spectacular scenery and geological importance.

Hopewell Rocks, Bay of Fundy (➤ 96)

Niagara Falls (➤ 44–45)

Parc Olympique (➤ 121)
The tower (175m/574ft) that rises over the Olympic Park gives wonderful views – up to 80km (50 miles) in clear weather.

Rocher Percé, Gaspésie (➤ 46–47)

Signal Hill, St. John's (➤ 50–51)

Sunsets over Lake Huron
Lake Huron is a very beautiful stretch of water, a gorgeous deep blue color. Watching the sun set across it on a fine evening is particularly magnificent, as are the occasional summer displays of the aurora borealis in the night sky. The Ontario shoreline both north and south of Goderich has some deserted stretches that are ideal for appreciating these phenomena. The observation tower at Parry Sound has a wonderful view over island-dotted Georgian Bay.

Great restaurants

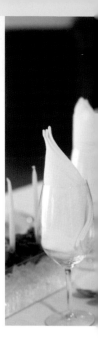

☗☗☗☗ The Cabot Club

Refined restaurant with a great view of Signal Hill
(► 50–51). The traditional Newfoundland dishes
include local seafood and wonderful desserts.

✉ The Fairmont Newfoundland, 115 Cavendish Square,
St. John's ☎ 709/726-4977; www.fairmont.com
🕒 Tue–Sat 6–10pm

☗☗ L'Express

Popular, unpretentious bistro with good seafood,
bouillabaisse, steak tartare and wonderful *frîtes* (fries).
Reservations essential.

✉ 3927 rue St-Denis, Montréal ☎ 514/845-5333 🕒 Mon–Fri
8am–2am, Sat–Sun 10am–1am

☗☗☗☗ North 44

Sophisticated restaurant with creative Continental
cuisine and impeccable service. Duck is a specialty.
Large wine list.

✉ 2537 Yonge Street, Toronto ☎ 416/487-4897;
www.north44restaurant.com 🕒 Mon–Sat 5–11

☗☗☗☗ Nuances

Gourmet French cuisine on the top floor of the casino. Great views
over the St. Lawrence River. Business attire.

✉ Pavillon de la France, 5th Floor, Casino du Montréal, 1 avenue du Casino,
Montréal ☎ 514/392-2708; 800/665-2274 ext 2708 (toll free);
www.casino-de-montreal.com 🕒 Daily 5:30–11pm (to 11:30pm Fri and Sat)

☗☗☗☗ Ryan Duffy's Steak and Seafood

This has been on top 100 Canadian restaurants list for more than
25 years. The dishes major on corn-fed steak and local seafood.

✉ 1650 Bedford Row, Halifax ☎ 902/421-1116; www.ryanduffys.ca
🕒 Mon–Fri 11:30–2, 5–10, Sat–Sun 5–10

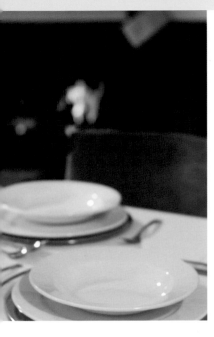

☙☙☙ Salty's on the Waterfront

The seafood is fresh and includes Atlantic salmon, lobster and mussels. Try to get a harbor view (➤ 84–85). ✉ 1869 Upper Water Street, Halifax ☎ 902/423-6818; www.saltys.ca ❸ Daily 11:30–10 (check seasonal variations)

☙☙☙☙ Signatures

The restaurant of Ottawa's Cordon Bleu Culinary Arts Institute is one of the highest rated in Canada. Based on traditional classic French cuisine, the food has inspired contemporary touches that make for an exciting menu.
✉ 453 Laurier Avenue East, Ottawa ☎ 888/289-6302 (toll free); 613/236-2460; www.restaurantsignatures.com ❸ Tue–Sat 5:30–10pm

☙☙☙☙☙ Truffles

In the Four Seasons Hotel and generally considered to be the best restaurant in town. Contemporary French menu in classy surroundings. Dress code: smart elegant, but jackets not required.
✉ Four Seasons Hotel, 21 Avenue Road, Toronto ☎ 416/964-0411; www.fourseasons.com ❸ Tue–Sat 6–10

☙☙ Wienstein and Gavino's Pasta Bar

A chic Italian eatery in the middle of the bar and nightclub district with lots of classic Italian main dishes and desserts.
✉ 1434 rue Crescent, Montréal ☎ 514/288-2231; www.wiensteinand gavinos.com ❸ Daily 11:30–11 (to midnight Thu–Sat), bar open until 3am

Great shopping

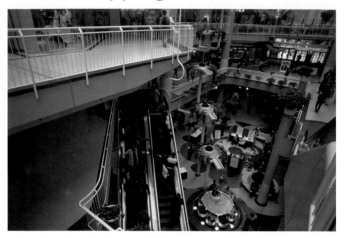

Bloor/Yorkville, Toronto

You can sniff affluence on the breeze in this corner of Toronto, where the city's wealthy flit between the designer boutiques and upscale galleries. The neighborhood includes the classy Hazelton Lanes mall. A great place to window shop and people-watch.

✉ Between Yonge, Bloor, Avenue and Davenport, Toronto, Ontario

Byward Market, Ottawa

This is Ottawa's most lively area, with a bustling street market where stands are piled high with fresh food, clothing and gifts. The surrounding streets are lined by specialty stores, boutiques and restaurants. The central market hall is also a venue for events.

✉ Byward Market Square and surrounding streets, Ottawa, Ontario

☎ 613/562-3325; www.byward-market.com 🕐 Daily

Champlain Place, Moncton

The second-biggest shopping mall in the Maritimes and the most central. It has more than 160 stores of all kinds, from the big three

(Sears, Wal-Mart and Sobeys) to fashion, sports and individual specialty stores. The Crystal Palace amusement complex is just across the parking lot.

✉ 477 Paul Street, Dieppe, Moncton, New Brunswick ☎ 506/867-0055; www.champlainplace.ca 🕓 Mon–Sat 10–9, Sun 12–5

Historic Properties, Halifax

In an area that's been a hive of activity for more than 250 years, this heritage district at the historic "Gateway to Canada" is now a great place for browsing (➤ 86–87).

✉ 1869 Upper Water Street, Halifax, Nova Scotia ☎ 902/429-0530; www.historicproperties.ca 🕓 Daily

Montréal Eaton Centre

Large shopping complex linked into the Underground City, with about 150 fashion stores and other retail outlets.

✉ 705 rue Ste-Catherine Ouest, Montréal, Québec ☎ 514/288-3708; http://centreeaton.shopping.ca 🕓 Mon–Fri 10–9, Sat 10–5, Sun 11–5 Ⓜ McGill

Quartier Petit Champlain, Québec City

In the historic heart of Québec City, this picturesque district is crammed full of enticing little boutiques selling fashions, crafts, art and jewelry, interspersed with cafés and restaurants.

✉ Lower Town, Québec City, Québec ☎ 418/692-2613; 877/692-2613 (toll free); www.quartierpetitchamplain.com 🕓 Mon–Sat 9:30–9, Sun 9:30–5

Toronto Eaton Centre

Probably Canada's most famous shopping destination, drawing around 50 million visitors a year. It's big, bright and airy and contains more than 250 stores of all kinds and several restaurants.

✉ 220 Yonge Street, between Dundas and Queen streets, Toronto, Ontario ☎ 416/598-8560; www.torontoeatoncentre.com 🕓 Mon–Fri 10–9, Sat 9:30–7, Sun 12–6 Ⓜ Dundas or Queen

Exploring

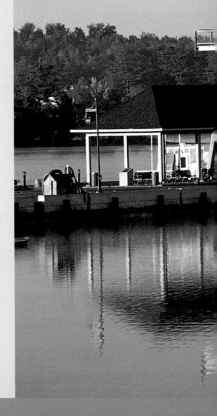

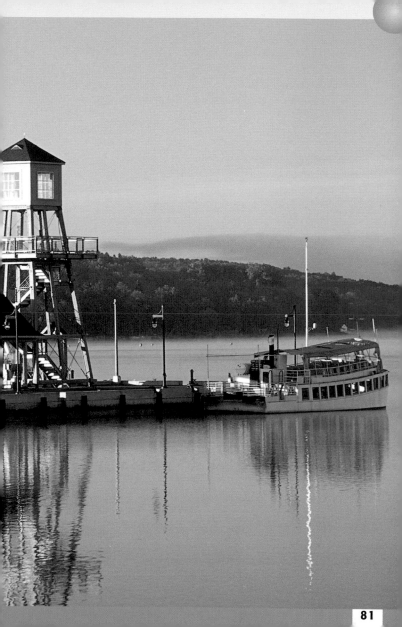

Eastern Canada consists of three regions: the Atlantic Provinces, Québec and Ontario. The culture is a blend of Acadian and Qúebecois French, Highland Scots and Irish, while Toronto is one of the most multicultural cities in the world. Here, too, are some historic towns and villages that date back to the earliest settlers, and fishing communities around the coast still land superb seafood.

The scenery in the east of the country matches that elsewhere and there are a number of national parks where you can enjoy the stunning landscape. The major cities are repositories of culture and have some of Canada's best museums.

Atlantic Provinces

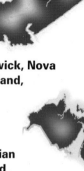

St John's

At the extreme eastern edge of Canada lie the provinces of New Brunswick, Nova Scotia, Prince Edward Island, and Newfoundland and Labrador. Steeped in the spray of the Atlantic Ocean, they are the smallest of all the Canadian provinces in both size and population.

Halifax

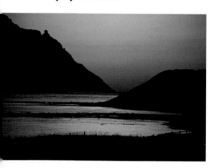

They are nevertheless strong in their traditional heritage, reflecting French Acadian roots, the earliest Loyalist settlements, the Gaelic culture of the Highland Scots and, in the case of Newfoundland, a strong Irish legacy. They boast major cities such as Halifax, Moncton and St. John's, charming communities like Charlottetown, Fredericton, St. Andrews-by-the-Sea, Lunenburg and Annapolis Royal, and the major historical restorations of Louisbourg and Village Historique Acadien. The scenery is amazingly varied, from the dramatic fjords of Gros Morne and the impressive seascapes of mountainous Cape Breton to the pretty rural landscape of Prince Edward Island and the fabulous tides of the Bay of Fundy.

HALIFAX

Everything in Halifax is marked by the sea. The waterfront is colorful, with a public walkway stretching for miles, while the city's streets are imbued with the ever-present salty feel and smell of the ocean.

Capital of Nova Scotia and the largest city of Atlantic Canada, Halifax is blessed with a magnificent natural harbor that extends nearly 16km (10 miles) inland. The outer harbor is divided from the Bedford Basin by a stretch called The Narrows, where the city climbs up a hill topped by a massive star-shaped fortress. The Citadel continues to dominate the town despite recent highrise construction.

Founded in July 1749, Halifax was from the start a military stronghold and naval base. During World War I, an event occurred that left a terrible mark on the city. In 1917, a French munitions ship, the *Mont Blanc*, had a fatal collision with a Belgian relief ship, the *Imo*, in The Narrows. What followed constituted the greatest man-made explosion the world had seen until the dropping of the atom bomb on Hiroshima in 1945. Not only was a huge area of the city destroyed and a large percentage of the population killed or injured, but even today it's impossible to visit the city without finding some reference to this tragedy.

Today, Halifax remains a naval place, home base for the Canadian Navy's Atlantic fleet, and is also an important commercial

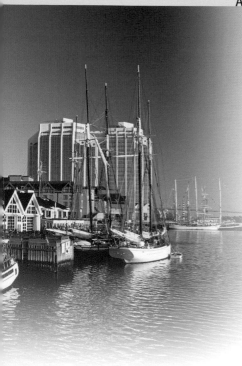

port with huge container terminals. Although the city sometimes suffers from fog and strong winds off the Atlantic, it is a fascinating place to visit - especially when the sun shines.
www.halifaxinfo.com
➕ 21H

Nova Scotia Visitors Centres
ℹ️ Scotia Square Visitor Centre, 5251 Duke Street, Halifax, Nova Scotia, B3J 1P3 ☎ 902/490-4000
🕐 Daily
ℹ️ Waterfront Visitor Centre, Sackville Landing, Halifax ☎ 902/490-4000

Art Gallery of Nova Scotia

Located in the heart of the city across the street from the Nova Scotia Legislature, this gallery occupies two 19th-century buildings connected by the Ondaatje Sculpture Court. The collection is made up of mainly Canadian works and the gallery hosts traveling exhibitions. A highlight is part of a house that once belonged to Maud Lewis, an artist from Digby, Nova Scotia, who decorated her home with colorful naive art.

www.artgalleryofnovascotia.ca
✉️ 1723 Hollis Street ☎ 902/424-7542 🕐 Daily 10–5 (to 9pm Thu)
🖐️ Moderate 🍴 Cheapside Café ($) ➤ 58 ❓ Guided tours daily 2:30 (Thu 2:30 and 7pm)

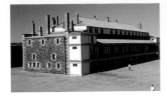

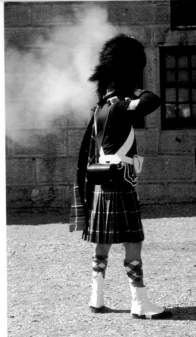

Citadel

Rising above the city, Citadel Hill offers fine views of its harbor and the bridges that span The Narrows to connect Halifax with Dartmouth on the opposite shore. Immediately below you is the Town Clock, a gift to the community from Prince Edward, father of Queen Victoria. The present Citadel, completed in 1865, is a national historic site. As you cross the drawbridge, you will meet staff posing as members of the 78th Highland Regiment, who were stationed here at that time. Wearing MacKenzie tartan kilts they will show you their barracks, guardroom, garrison cell and powder magazine. Each day they fire the noon gun, by which everyone in Halifax sets their clocks.

www.pc.gc.ca/lhn-nhs/ns/halifax

✉ Corner of Sackville and Brunswick streets ☎ 902/426-508 🕔 Early May–Oct 9–5 (to 6pm Jul–Aug); Nov–early May grounds only open ✋ Moderate 🍴 Coffee shop ($) ❓ Regimental gift store. Military drills. Guided tours

Historic Properties

In the 1970s, a number of 19th-century waterfront warehouses were renovated. Known as Historic Properties, they now house craft stores, an excellent food market and several restaurants.

If you walk along the waterfront walkway (4km/2.5 miles) you can visit, among other attractions, the Maritime Museum of the Atlantic (➤ 88), the *Bluenose II* (if she is visiting; ➤ 99) and the ferry to Dartmouth. Beyond the new complexes is Pier 21 which was the entry point to Canada for over a million immigrants between 1928 and 1971, and is now an award-winning musuem.
www.historicproperties.ca

✉ Upper Water Street ☎ 902/429-0530 ✋ Free. Parking: expensive
🍴 Food market and variety of restaurants ($–$$)

Pier 21 National Historic Site

✉ 1055 Marginal Road ☎ 902/425-7770; www.pier21.ca ⏱ May–late
Nov daily 9:30–5:30; late Nov–Apr; Tue–Sat 10–5, (also Mon in Apr)
✋ Moderate 🍴 Café ($)

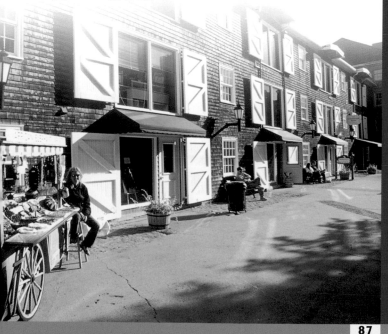

Maritime Museum of the Atlantic

On the waterfront, partly located in the former William Robertson ship's chandlery, this maritime museum boasts a number of full-size ships floating beside it as well as a model collection inside. There are fascinating displays about the *Titanic* (many of the unidentified bodies were buried in Halifax) and the Halifax Explosion (► 84). There is also a section devoted to the Cunard Steamship Line, because Samuel Cunard, its founder, was from Halifax. The highlight is probably the restored ship's chandlery of 1879, complete with owner William Robertson behind the counter.

During the summer, you can explore the HMCS *Sackville*, the sole survivor of more than 100 corvettes that were built in Canada to escort convoys across the Atlantic during World War II.

http://museum.gov.ns.ca/mma

✉ 1675 Lower Water Street ☎ 902/424-7490 ☻ May–Oct daily 9:30–5:30 (to 8pm Tue; closed Sun am May and Oct); Nov–Apr Tue 9:30–8, Wed–Sat 9:30–5, Sun 1–5. HMCS *Sackville*: daily, Jun–Sep 👌 Moderate; small additional fee for HMCS *Sackville* 🍴 Restaurants nearby ($–$$)

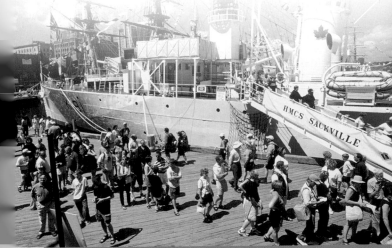

More to see in the Atlantic Provinces

ANNAPOLIS ROYAL

Twice daily, the great tides of the Bay of Fundy rush into the Annapolis Basin, reversing the flow of the river at tiny Annapolis Royal and providing electricity through North America's only tidal power generating station.

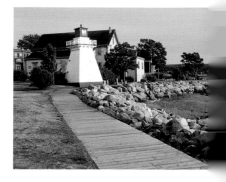

Today, the town is a gracious mixture of heritage and charm, and its main street is lined by elegant homes, craft shops, art galleries and restaurants. Once, however, it was the most fought over place in Canada, changing hands frequently between the English and the French. In the center of the community is **Fort Anne,** whose picturesque site offers sweeping views of the Annapolis Basin from its well-preserved earthworks. A short drive 10.5km (6.5 miles) west takes you to **Port Royal,** founded in 1605 by Samuel de Champlain, making it the first French colony on the continent. The reconstructed wooden buildings form a distinctive compound and contain both working and living areas.

www.annapolisroyal.com

✚ 20G ✉ 236 Prince Albert Road, Box 2, Annapolis Royal, Nova Scotia
☎ 902/532-5454

Fort Anne and Port Royal National Historic Sites

✉ P.O. Box 9, Annapolis Royal, Nova Scotia, B0S 1A0 ☎ 902/532-2397; 902/532-2321 (off season); www.pc.gc.ca/lhn-nhs/ns/fortanne; www.pc.gc.ca/lhn-nhs/ns/portroyal ❹ Mid-May to mid-Oct daily 9–5:30 (to 6pm Jul–Aug) ⚇ Inexpensive ❙❙ Restaurants in Annapolis Royal ($–$$)

AVALON PENINSULA

On the east coast of Newfoundland, the Avalon Peninsula seems to hang suspended from the rest of the island by a narrow isthmus. At longitude 52° 37′ 24″ and latitude 47° 31′ 17″, **Cape Spear** (southeast of St. John's) is the most easterly point of the entire North American continent. Today, it is a national historic park and the lighthouse can be visited. Elsewhere along the peninsula, the coastline is ruggedly beautiful. At St. Vincent's, the deep water allows whales to come close to shore. Bird Rock, off Cape St. Mary's, has colonies of northern gannets, razorbills and murres, while at Witless Bay, huge icebergs can be seen in early summer, along with more whales and seabirds.

✚ 23L ❓ Witless Bay is 31km (19 miles) south of St. John's via Route 10. Cape St. Mary's is 102km (63 miles) south of the Trans-Canada Highway via Route 90. St. Vincent's is 80km (50 miles) south of the Trans-Canada Highway via Route 90.

Cape Spear National Historic Site

✉ P.O. Box 1268, St. John's, Newfoundland and Labrador, A1C 5M9 ☎ 709/772-5367; www.pc.gc.ca/lhn-nhs/nl/spear

🕒 Grounds: daily. Visitor center: mid-May to Labour Day daily 8:30–9, then 10–6 until mid-Oct. Lighthouse: mid-May to mid-Oct daily 10–6

✋ Inexpensive 🍴 Restaurants in St. John's ❓ 11km (7 miles) from St. John's via Route 11

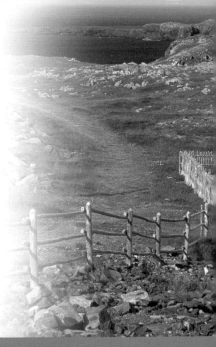

BONAVISTA PENINSULA

On Newfoundland's east coast is the Bonavista Peninsula, which is dotted with a number of picturesque communities. The tiny village of Trinity was once a prosperous fishing center and a lot of its charm remains. Colorful Newfoundland "box" houses are set on a hilly peninsula that has fine views of the ocean and the small protected harbor. Bonavista is another tranquil community, best known for its rocky cape where John Cabot is supposed to have made his first North American landfall.

✚ 23M 🍴 Restaurants in Trinity and Bonavista ($–$$) ❓ Trinity is 74km (46 miles) and Bonavista is 114km (71 miles) from the Trans-Canada Highway at Clarenville via Route 230. Cape Bonavista is 5km (3 miles) from Bonavista

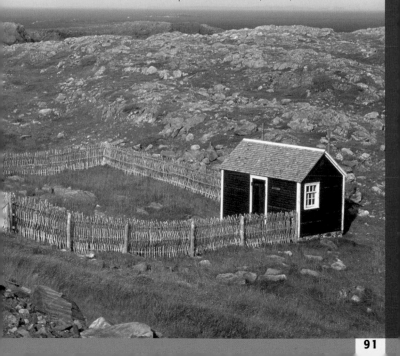

CAMPOBELLO ISLAND

Set at the point where the Atlantic Ocean floods into the Bay of Fundy, Campobello Island has long been famous for its invigorating climate. In the late 19th century, wealthy industrialists built summer homes here, among them the parents of Franklin Delano Roosevelt, U.S. president in 1933–45. Roosevelt and his wife had their own summer "cottage" on the island, which is today the centerpiece of an **international peace park.**

www.campobello.com

✚ 12E   ℹ️ Campobello Island Visitor Center

☎ 506/752-7043

Roosevelt-Campobello International Park

✉ 459 Route 774, Welshpool ☎ 506/752-2922; www.fdr.net ⏰ Mid-May to mid-Oct daily 10–6 ✋ Free

FREDERICTON

New Brunswick's capital is a quiet, pretty city of elm-lined streets set on a wide bend of the St. John River. The excellent **Beaverbrook Art Gallery,** has an outstanding collection of British paintings. About 34km (21 miles) west of the city is **Kings Landing** historical settlement, a fascinating recreation of 19th-century Loyalist life set on a fine site in the St. John valley.

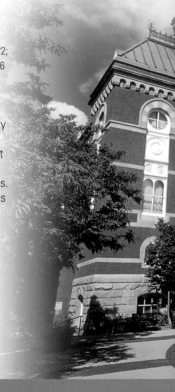

www.city.fredericton.nb.ca

✚ 19H   ✉ 11 Carleton Street

☎ 506/460-2041; 888/888-4768 (toll free)

Beaverbrook Art Gallery

✉ 703 Queen Street ☎ 506/458-2028; www.beaverbrookartgallery.org

⏰ Daily 9–5:30 (to 9pm Thu) ✋ Moderate

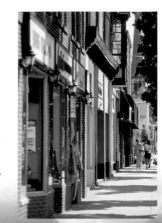

Kings Landing

✉ 20 Kings Landing Road, Kings Landing; exit 253 of TCH ☎ 506/363-4999; 506/363-4959 (recorded information); www.kingslanding.nb.ca

🕐 Early Jun to mid-Oct daily 10–5

✋ Expensive 🍴 King's Head Inn ($$), café ($), ice-cream parlor

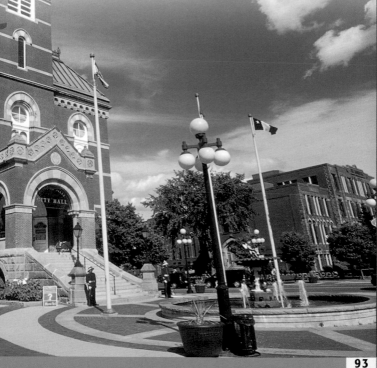

FUNDY ISLANDS

Deer, Grand Manan and Campobello (➤ 92) islands are located in the mouth of Passamaquoddy Bay, geographically closer to Maine, U.S.A. than to Canada. The high tides and currents of the bay act as giant nutrient pumps that lure all kinds of creatures, from herring and tuna to whales. People visit the islands for a quiet retreat, to watch birds and to view whales.

www.grandmanannb.com

www.deerisland.nb.ca

✚ 12E 🛈 Grand Manan Tourist Association and Chamber of Commerce ☎ 506/662-3442; 888/525-1655 (toll free)
🚢 Deer Island ferry daily from L'Etete, New Brunswick (☎ 888/747-7006); Grand Manan ferry daily from Blacks Harbour, New Brunswick (☎ 506/662-3724)

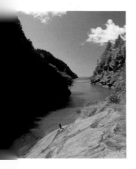

FUNDY NATIONAL PARK

On the Bay of Fundy, this park is a wonderful combination of coastal highlands and shoreline. The bay, with its vast tidal range and cold water, influences the entire park. You can experience this tidal fluctuation on the bay's shores by watching fishing boats come and go. At Alma, it takes less than an hour for the water to go from nothing to waist-deep.

www.pc.gc.ca/pn-np/nb/fundy

✚ 20H ✉ P.O. Box 1001, Alma, New Brunswick, E4H 1B4
☎ 506/887-6000 🕐 Daily (reception center closed weekends in winter) 🖐 Moderate 🍴 Restaurants, Alma ($–$$)

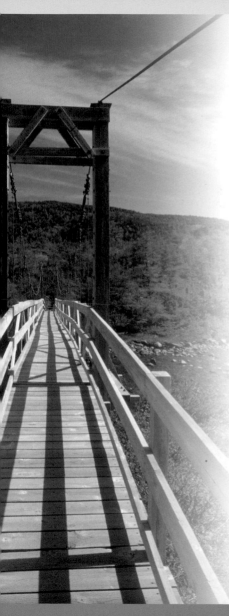

GROS MORNE NATIONAL PARK

On Newfoundland's west coast is Gros Morne, a spectacularly wild area of fjords, sea coast, forest and mountains. In 1987 it was designated a World Heritage Site by UNESCO for the international importance of its geological features. The Gros Morne Tablelands consist of peridotite from the Earth's mantle. Formed some 450 million years ago, these ocher-colored rocks are an incredibly rare occurrence at the Earth's surface. A visit to the Park Discovery Centre in Woody Point, overlooking beautiful Bonne Bay, offers an excellent introduction.

www.pc.gc.ca/pn-np/nl/grosmorne

✚ 21L ✉ P.O. Box 130, Rocky Harbour, Newfoundland and Labrador, A0K 4N0

☎ 709/458-2417 ⓭ Daily 🖐 Moderate 🍴 Food services in Rocky Harbour and Woody Point ($–$$)

HOPEWELL ROCKS

There is nowhere better than this to experience the highest tides in the world. Come at low tide and you can walk on the beach beneath these rocky columns, some rising to more than 16m (52ft) and topped by trees. Return at high tide and they appear as tiny islands in the bay. Check tide tables carefully before descending to the beach – the water rushes in very quickly. An Interpretive Centre (mid-May to mid-Oct daily) explains the phenomenon.

🕇 20H ✉ Located 40km (25 miles south of Moncton on Highway 114)
🕐 Daily (when parking lot is closed, walk from approach road)
🅿 Parking: moderate 🍴 Food service ($), picnic area

L'ANSE AUX MEADOWS

Christopher Columbus and John Cabot have gone down in history as the great "discoverers" of North America. This site proves they were beaten to it some 400 years earlier by Vikings. It is thought the Vikings came here seasonally to fish and collect fruit to take back to Scandinavia and for expeditions to mainland Canada. Three buildings have been reconstructed and there's an exhibition and a collection of objects excavated at this UNESCO World Heritage Site.
www.pc.gc.ca/lhn-nhs/meadows

🕇 21M ✉ P.O. Box 70, St. Lunaire-Griquet, Newfoundland and Labrador, A0K 2X0 ☎ 709/623-2608 🕐 Jun–early Oct daily 9–6
🅿 Moderate 🍴 Restaurants in St. Anthony, 40km (25 miles away)

LABRADOR

Towering mountains, huge lakes and fast-flowing rivers make Labrador one of the world's few remaining wilderness areas and much of the region is inaccessible. A ferry from St. Barbe on Newfoundland to Blanc Sablon in Québec enables you to access the Labrador coast and drive up it for a short distance, or you can drive Route 389 from Baie Comeau in Québec to Labrador City.

Red Bay (78km/48 miles from the ferry) was the whaling capital of the world in the 16th century. Dozens of Basque fishermen came here to hunt whales in order to supply Europe with oil for lamps and soap. An interpretation center recreates these times.
www.newfoundlandandlabradortourism.com

✠ 18M ℹ Newfoundland and Labrador Department of Tourism, P.O. Box 8700, St. John's, Newfoundland and Labrador, A1B 4J6 ☎ 709/729-0862; 800/563-6353 (toll free)

Red Bay National Historic Site

✉ P.O. Box 103, Red Bay, Newfoundland and Labrador, A0K 4K0 ☎ 709/920-2142; www.pc.gc.ca/lhn-nhs/nl/redbay ⏱ Early Jun–early Oct daily 9–6 ✋ Moderate

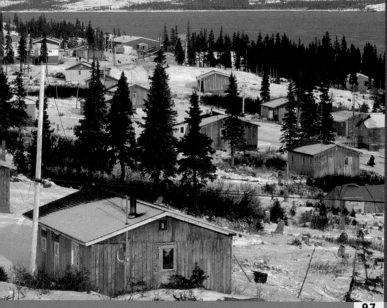

LOUISBOURG

At one time, Louisbourg was the great fortress of New France,
guarding the St. Lawrence River and the colony. Constructed in the
early 18th century, it had the largest garrison in North America.
Captured and destroyed by the British in 1758, the fort lay in ruins
for two centuries, but today it has risen from the ashes. Covering
4.8ha (12 acres), the site now holds a faithful recreation of a town
of the 1740s. From the visitor center you can walk or take a shuttle
bus to the entrance. The 50-plus buildings, of wood or roughcast
masonry are furnished in 1740s style and populated with suitably
attired "residents." Tour the King's
Bastion and visit the governor's
apartments, and don't miss
the barracks, where soldiers
will regale you with stories of
their everyday lives.

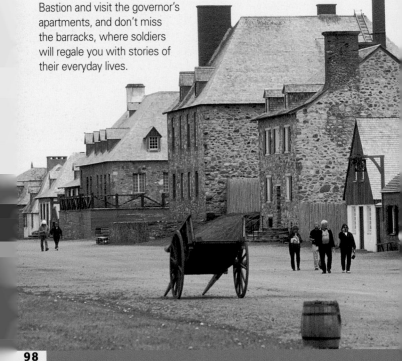

www.pc.gc.ca/lhn-nhs/ns/louisbourg

✚ 22J ✉ 259 Park Service Road, Louisbourg, Nova Scotia, B1C 2L2

☎ 902/733-2280 🕓 Jul–Aug daily 9–5:30; mid-May to Jun and Sep to mid-Oct daily 9:30–5; early May and mid- to late Oct daily 9:30–5, (no animation and limited access to buildings); closed Nov–Apr ✋ Expensive

🍴 Restaurants ($–$$) ❓ Craft demonstrations, military drills, etc

LUNENBURG

Set on a hillside and characterized by narrow streets and wood-framed buildings, Lunenburg radiates the flavor of its seafaring heritage. A UNESCO World Heritage Site since 1995, it has a waterfront active with the fishing and shipbuilding industries that have been the backbone of its prosperity since its foundation in 1753. The bright red buildings of the **Fisheries Museum**

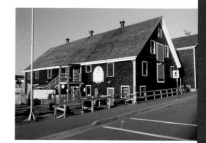

of the Atlantic commemorate this heritage, and offer interesting displays and activities. In summer, the schooner *Bluenose II* is often in the port. Visitors can board the boat for a trip.

www.explorelunenburg.ca

✚ 21G ✉ Blockhouse Road ☎ 902/634-8100

Fisheries Museum of the Atlantic

✉ 68 Bluenose Drive ☎ 902/634-4794; 866/579-4909 (toll free); http://museum.gov.ns.ca/fma 🕓 May–Oct daily 9:30–5:30 (to 7pm Tue–Sat Jul–Aug); Nov–Apr Mon–Fri 9:30–4, but closed holidays ✋ Moderate (Nov to mid-Mar inexpensive) 🍴 Old Fish Factory ($$) (☎ 902/634-3333)

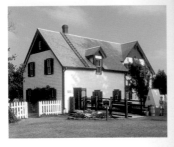

PRINCE EDWARD ISLAND

Tiny Prince Edward Island (known as PEI) has quiet rural landscapes, bright red soil and fine sandy beaches and is connected to the mainland by Confederation Bridge. PEI is known worldwide as the setting for Lucy Maud Montgomery's classic tale of redheaded orphan, *Anne of Green Gables* and fans of the book shouldn't miss visiting period-furnished **Green Gables House.**

The island's capital, Charlottetown, is a delightful place to saunter around. It was the birthplace of Canada, following a meeting of colonial movers and shakers who came to discuss confederation in 1864 in the stately Province House. **Founders Hall,** with costumed guides, traces the country's history.

www.gov.pe.ca

➕ 20H ✉ Box 940, Charlottetown, Prince Edward Island, C1A 7M5
☎ 902/368-4444; 800/463-4734 (toll free)

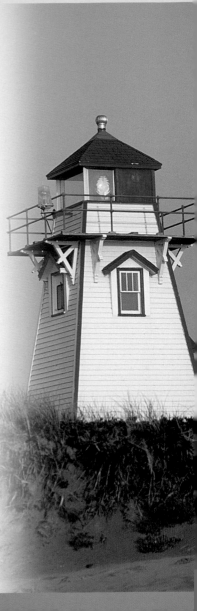

Charlottetown Visitor Centre ✉ 6 Prince Street ☎ 902 368-6613; 800/463-4PEI (toll-free)

Green Gables House ✉ Route 6, Cavendish, Prince Edward Island National Park ☎ 902/963-7874; www.pc.gc.ca/lhn-nhs/pe/greengables ③ Jul–late Aug daily 9–6 (to 8pm Tue and Thu); May–Jun and late Aug–Oct daily 9–5; Apr and Nov–late Dec Sun–Thu 10–4; early Jan–Mar Sun–Thu noon–4. Closed Easter ⚲ Moderate 🍴 Café ($)

Founders Hall ✉ 6 Prince Street, Charlottetown ☎ 902/368-1864; 800/955-1864 (toll free); www.foundershall.ca ③ Mid-May to early Oct daily; early Oct–Nov and Feb to mid-May Tue–Sat. Closed Dec–Jan ⚲ Moderate

ST. ANDREWS-BY-THE-SEA

Right at the end of a peninsula extending into Passamaquoddy Bay, St. Andrews-by-the-Sea is a small community and a National Historic District. It was settled by Loyalists in 1783, and its tree-lined streets are named after King George III's 15 children. Later, St. Andrews became a fashionable place for the wealthy to build summer homes.

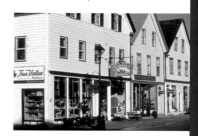

The town has many attractions, including the **Huntsman Marine Science Centre** but find time to stroll the quaint streets and admire the Georgian houses as well.

www.townofstandrews.ca; **www.**townsearch.com/standrews
✚ 12E 🛈 St. Andrews Chamber of Commerce: 46 Reed Avenue, St. Andrews-by-the-Sea, New Brunswick, E5B 1A1 ☎ 506/529-3555; 800/563-7397 (toll free)

Huntsman Marine Science Centre
✉ 1 Lower Campus Road ☎ 506/529-1200; www.huntsmanmarine.ca
③ Late May–early Sep daily 10–5; early Sep–late May Thu–Sun 10–5 (seal feeding times 11am and 4pm) ⚲ Moderate

ST. JOHN'S

Facing the open Atlantic in the extreme east of
Newfoundland, the province's capital has a spectacular site on
the slopes of a natural harbor. The steep streets are a clutter
of colorful wooden houses and the harbor is full of the ships

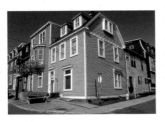

of many nations. St. John's
inhabitants, many of Irish
descent, have a distinctive
accent and a great sense
of humor; and they adore
their city.

One downtown
landmark that's hard to
miss is **The Rooms,** a
brightly painted structure resembling a giant group of the old
fish processing "rooms". It's Newfoundland's premier cultural
center, containing the provincial museum, art gallery and archives,
artists in residence, a multimedia theater and performance space.

From the harbor, there are boat trips to view whales and the
summer icebergs. Peek inside the Murray Premises Hotel,
renovated 1846 fishing warehouses (➤ 106), and on the road to
Signal Hill (➤ 50–51) note the entrance to the **Johnson Geo
Centre,** a great geological showcase constructed underground.
www.stjohns.ca

✚ 23L ⓘ City Hall 1st Floor, 35 New Gower Street, St. John's,
Newfoundland and Labrador, A1C 5M2 ☎ 709/576-8106

The Rooms

✉ 9 Bonaventure Avenue ☎ 709/757 8000; www.therooms.ca ⊕ Jun to
mid-Oct Mon–Sat 10–5 (to 9pm Wed), Sun noon–5; mid-Oct to May Tue–Sat
10–5 (to 9pm Wed and Thu), Sun noon–5 💰 Moderate (free Wed 6–9pm)

Johnson Geo Centre

✉ 175 Signal Hill Road ☎ 709/737-7880; 866/868-7625 (toll free);
www.geocentre.ca ⊕ Mon–Sat 9:30–5, Sun noon–5; closed Mon mid-Oct
to mid-May 💰 Moderate ❓ Geo-boutique with geological items

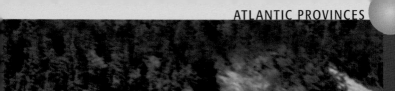

TERRA NOVA NATIONAL PARK

At Terra Nova, on the east coast of Newfoundland, forested hills rise above a rocky, fjord-like coastline, creating an area rich in wildlife and scenic beauty. Moose, lynx and black bear haunt the forests, bald eagles and great horned owls soar overhead, and whales and other marine life frequent the waters offshore.

Terra Nova is easily accessible, since the Trans-Canada Highway

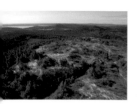

bisects it. Most park facilities are located on Newman Sound, including the Marine Interpretation Centre in Saltons. There are also boat tours, which provide opportunities for observing different aspects of the life of the Sound, and several viewpoints on land.

www.pc.gc.ca/pn-np/nl/terranova

✚ 23M ✉ Glovertown, Newfoundland and Labrador, A0G 2L0. 240km (149 miles) from St. John's ☎ 709/533-28001 ⏰ Daily (visitor center closed Tue–Wed early Jan–late Apr) 🐾 Moderate ⛴ For boat tours on Newman Sound, contact Ocean Watch Tours (☎ 709/533-6024)

VILLAGE HISTORIQUE ACADIEN

Located on New Brunswick's Acadian Peninsula, this recreated village provides an authentic representation of French Acadian life between 1770 and 1939. The story of the Acadians is a sad one. Expelled from their farmlands in Nova Scotia in 1755, most of these settlers were deported to the southern British colonies. Eventually some made their way north again to settle in this area.

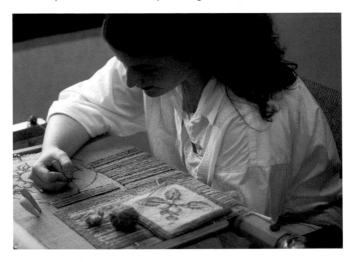

Interpreters in period costume bring the place to life, and visitors can explore the 40 buildings and watch displays to discover more about Acadian customs and trades.

www.villagehistoriqueacadien.com

🕂 19J 🖂 14311 Road 11, P.O. Box 5626, Caraquet, New Brunswick, E1W 1B7. 10km (6 miles) west of Caraquet in northeastern New Brunswick
☎ 506/726-2600; 877/721-2200 (toll free) 🕓 Early Jun to mid-Sep daily 10–6; mid-Sep to late Sep daily 10–5 (5 buildings open) 🖐 Expensive
🍴 Restaurant and food services ($–$$) ❓ Store selling Acadian items

HOTELS

CHARLOTTETOWN, PRINCE EDWARD ISLAND
♦♦♦ The Great George ($$$)
This inn has several properties, providing luxury accommodations in 19th-century style. Some rooms have fireplace and Jacuzzi, and all are elegantly furnished with antiques. Breakfast included.
✉ 58 Great George Street ☎ 902/892-0606; 800/361-1118 (toll free); www.thegreatgeorge.com

CHÉTICAMP
♦♦ Cabot Trail Sea and Golf Chalets ($$)
Just outside the Cape Breton Highlands National Park, this complex offers one- or two-bedroom housekeeping chalets. A private path leads to the golf course.
✉ 71 Fraser Doucet Lane, PO Box 324 ☎ 902/224-1777; 877/244-1777 (toll free); www.seagolfchalets.com

FREDERICTON, NEW BRUNSWICK
♦♦♦ Crowne Plaza Fredericton Lord Beaverbrook Hotel ($$$)
Elegant hotel with unbeatable location downtown near the Legislative Assembly and Beaverbrook Art Gallery (➤ 92). The Terrace restaurant overlooks the St. John River.
✉ 659 Queen Street ☎ 506/455-3371; 877/579-7666 (toll free); www.cpfredericton.com

HALIFAX
♦♦♦ Waverley Inn ($$)
Historic bed-and-breakfast, with hardwood floors and fine antique furniture, in a peaceful area close to downtown.
✉ 1266 Barrington Street ☎ 902/423-9346; 800/565-9346; www.waverleyinn.com

NORTH RUSTICO, PRINCE EDWARD ISLAND
♦♦ Gulf View Cottages ($$)
Fully equipped two-bedroom cottages with a fine site overlooking the Gulf of St. Lawrence in Prince Edward Island National Park. Cycling and jogging trails; beach.

✉ Gulf Shore Road ☎ 902/963-2052; 877/963-2052 (toll free); www.gulfviewcottages.com ⏰ Closed early-Oct to late-May

ST. JOHN'S, NEWFOUNDLAND
▼▼▼ Murray Premises Hotel ($$$)

Former warehouse overlooking the harbor, restored as a luxurious boutique hotel. Old beams and exposed brickwork beautifully set off the up-to-the-minute facilities. Two restaurants.

✉ 5 Becks Cove ☎ 709/738-7773; 866/738-7773 (toll free); www.murraypremiseshotel.com

RESTAURANTS

ANNAPOLIS ROYAL, NOVA SCOTIA
▼▼▼ Garrison House Dining Room ($$)

In a 19th-century house opposite Fort Anne (➤ 89). Good food in small intimate dining rooms. Seafood specialties.

✉ 350 St. George Street ☎ 902/532-5750; 866/532-5750; www.garrison house.ca ⏰ Early May to mid-Dec daily 5–8 (to 9pm high season)

CHARLOTTETOWN, PRINCE EDWARD ISLAND
▼▼ Chez Cora ($–$$)

This Québec-based breakfast-and-lunch chain is going from strength to strength. They serve a terrific range of good healthy food (fresh fruit with everything) and deliciously naughty treats.

✉ 476 Queen Street ☎ 506/472-2672; www.chezcora.com

▼▼ Gahan House ($–$$)

Traditional brew-pub with above-average food, including fish and chips coated in batter made with the brewery's own ale.

✉ 126 Sydney Street ☎ 902/626-2337; www.gahan.ca ⏰ Mon–Thu 11–11, Fri–Sat 11am–1am, Sun 11–9 (kitchen closes one hour before closing time)

DIEPPE, NEW BRUNSWICK
▼▼▼ L'Idylle ($$–$$$)

An elegant restaurant in an 1828 home, where owner/chef Emmanuel Charretier and his wife, both from France, serve authentic French cuisine (and grow many of the vegetables and fruits).

✉ 1788 Amirault Street ☎ 506/860-6641; www.restaurantidylle.com
🕓 Mon–Sat 5–10pm

FREDERICTON, NEW BRUNSWICK
🍷🍷 Brewbakers ($$)

Seafood, crispy pizza from the wood-fired oven and interesting salads are served in a warren of rooms as well as on an outdoor patio and in the bar.

✉ 546 King Street ☎ 506/459-0067; www.brewbakers.ca 🕓 Mon–Thu 11:30–10, Fri 11:30–11, Sat 4–11, Sun 4–10

SAINT JOHN, NEW BRUNSWICK
🍷🍷 Steamers Lobster Company ($$–$$$)

There's lobster, of course, in this restaurant specializing in market-fresh local seafood. There are also meat choices such as prime rib and stir fries. Dinner theater some nights.

✉ 110 Water Street ☎ 506/648-2325; www.steamerslobstercompany.com
🕓 Daily 4–10

HALIFAX, NOVA SCOTIA
🍷🍷🍷 McKelvie's Delishes Fishes Dishes ($–$$)

In a refurbished firehouse with an outdoor patio in the summer months. A great place for seafood, pasta, chowders, and desserts.

✉ 1680 Lower Water Street ☎ 902/421-6161; www.mckelvies.com
🕓 Mon–Sat 11:30–10, Sun 4:30–10

🍷🍷🍷 Salty's on the Waterfront ($$–$$$)

See page 77.

MOBILE, NEWFOUNDLAND
🍷🍷 Captain's Table ($$)

Named after Captain William Jackman, a Newfoundland hero. Great seafood, chowder and other traditional Newfoundland dishes. Pleasant dining room with open fireplace.

✉ Mobile ☎ 709/334-2278; www.captainstable.nf.ca 🕓 Daily 11:30–9; Oct 1–Apr 30 Wed–Sun noon–8

ST. JOHN'S, NEWFOUNDLAND
WWW The Cellar ($$–$$$)
Fine dining with some local dishes and an extensive wine list.
⊠ 189 Water Street ☎ 709/579-8900; www.thecellarrestaurant.ca
🕔 Mon–Fri 11:30–2:30, 5:30–9:30 (10pm Fri), Sat 5:30–10, Sun 5:30–9:30

SUMMERSIDE, PRINCE EDWARD ISLAND
WW Starlite Diner ($)
A 1950s-style diner, complete with jukeboxes in the booths.
Home-style cooking, including fried clams, burgers, barbecued
chicken, hot dogs and great desserts.
⊠ 810 Water Street ☎ 902/436-7752; www.starlitediner.pe.ca

SHOPPING

SHOPPING CENTERS AND MALLS
Avalon Mall
Northwest of the city. Attractive mall on two levels, with 140
stores, including clothing, books, music, gifts and jewelry stores,
Sobeys supermarket and Wal-Mart. Large movie theater complex;
food court and restaurants.
⊠ 48 Kenmount Road, St. John's, Newfoundland ☎ 709/753-7144;
www.shopavalonmall.com 🕔 Mon–Sat 10–10, Sun 12–5

Champlain Place
See pages 78–79.

Halifax Shopping Centre
To the west of downtown. Biggest mall in the Maritimes, with
over 170 stores, including boutiques, sports stores, pharmacies,
banks, Sears and Wal-Mart. Fast-food outlets.
⊠ 7001 Mumford Road, Halifax, Nova Scotia ☎ 902/453-1752;
www.halifaxshoppingcentre.com 🕔 Mon–Sat 9:30–9; Sun noon–5

MARKETS
Boyce Farmers' Market
About 200 vendors sell local produce, crafts and gifts at this
longtime institution in downtown.

✉ 665 George Street, Fredericton, New Brunswick ☎ 506/451-1815; www.boycefarmersmarket.com ⏰ Sat 6am–1pm

Halifax Farmers' Market
In the courtyards of a former brewery, this market is a hive of activity on Saturdays. Relocating to a spectacular new location on the waterfront, when it will operate six days a week.

✉ Keith's Brewery Building, 1496 Lower Water Street (moving to Pier 20), Halifax, Nova Scotia ☎ 902/492-4043; http://halifaxfarmersmarket.com ⏰ Sat 7am–1pm

CRAFTS, ANTIQUES AND OTHER SPECIALTIES
Great Village Antiques Marketplace
This is Nova Scotia's biggest antiques market, with 18 specialist dealers. China, glass, furniture, folk art, toys, jewelry, and more.

✉ 8728 Highway 2, Great Village (northwest of Truro, off Trans-Canada Highway), Nova Scotia ☎ 902/668-2149; www.greatvillageantiques.com ⏰ Mar–Dec Mon–Sat 10–5, Sun 1–5

River Valley Crafts and Artisan Gift Shops
A number of craftspeople sell their wares such as painting, jewelry, First Nations crafts and Celtic art on the main floor of the former Soldiers' Barracks in downtown's historic Garrison district.

✉ Barracks Square, Carleton Street, Fredericton, New Brunswick ☎ 506/460-2837; 888/888-4768 ⏰ Closed Oct–May

ENTERTAINMENT

CHILDREN'S ENTERTAINMENT
Fluvarium
Windows below water level show the life of a real stream full of trout, frogs and tadpoles. Feeding time 4pm.

✉ Nagles Place, Pippy Park, St. John's, Newfoundland ☎ 709/754-3474; www.fluvarium.ca ⏰ Mon–Fri 9–5, Sat–Sun 12–5 💲 Inexpensive

Science East
More than 100 exhibits. Children can step inside a huge kaleido-scope or see their hair stand on end in the static electricity display.

✉ 668 Brunswick Street, Fredericton, New Brunswick ☎ 506/457-2340;
www.scienceeast.nb.ca 🕐 Jun–Aug Mon–Sat 10–5, Sun 1–4; Sep–May
Mon–Fri 12–5, Sat 10–5 💷 Inexpensive

THEATERS AND NIGHTCLUBS
Grafton Street Dinner Theatre
Specializes in lighthearted musical comedies served up during
dinner by staff in costume. Audience participation encouraged.
✉ 1741 Grafton Street, Halifax, Nova Scotia ☎ 902/425-1961;
www.graftonstdinnertheatre.com

King's Theatre
Live theater, concerts and movies presented year-round in a
historic building on the town's main street. Also a summer festival.
✉ 209 St. George Street, Annapolis Royal, Nova Scotia ☎ 902/532-7704;
902/532-5466 (24-hour listings); www.kingstheatre.ca

Neptune
Famous Canadian theater company presenting drama, music and
comedy in two auditoriums year-round.
✉ 1593 Argyle Street, Halifax, Nova Scotia ☎ 902/429-7070; 800/565-7345
(toll free); www.neptunetheatre.com

Olde Dublin Pub
Irish pub open year-round, with live entertainment and traditional
music on Saturdays and Sundays, May–September.
✉ 131 Sydney Street, Charlottetown, Prince Edward Island
☎ 902/892-6992; www.oldedublinpub.com

The Playhouse
Next to the Provincial Legislature. Theater presenting drama,
comedy and all kinds of musical performances year-round.
✉ 686 Queen Street, Fredericton, New Brunswick ☎ 506/458-8344;
866/884-5800 (toll free); www.theplayhouse.nb.ca

Québec

The heart of French Canada, the province of Québec is simply gigantic, extending 1,900km (1,200 miles) north from the U.S. border to the shores of the Hudson Strait. A land of sharp contrasts, it is resolutely distinct in its culture and lifestyle.

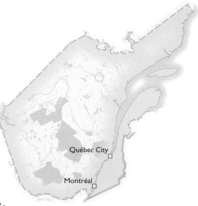

Québec City

Montréal

Traversed by the magnificent St. Lawrence, one of the world's

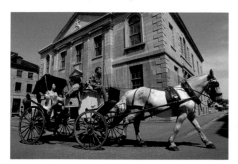

great rivers, Québec boasts some spectacular scenery. The Gaspé Peninsula has awe-inspiring seascapes, Saguenay Fjord is bounded by impressive cliffs and filled with dark waters, and the Charlevoix coast offers sweeping views of river and hinterland. Elsewhere, visitors can enjoy the tranquility of the Eastern Townships or the bustling sports-oriented ambience of the Laurentians. Add to these cosmopolitan, sophisticated Montréal, with its great restaurants and summer festivals, and the old-world charm of the capital, Québec City, and the great diversity of the province can be fully appreciated.

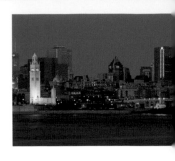

MONTRÉAL

Montréal is urbane, sophisticated and cosmopolitan. Although this is the second-largest French-speaking city in the world, fully one-third of the population is non-French, giving it a tremendous cultural vitality.

In 1642, Ville-Marie de Montréal was founded as a Roman Catholic mission; even a hundred years ago it was dominated by the towers and spires of its churches, gaining it the moniker "the city of one hundred steeples." This religious heritage is still evident in the city's churches, even though they stand empty today. It is also evident in the cross on top of Mont-Royal, illuminated at night.

In 1760, the British conquered the city and the economy became the domain of a group of industrious Scots. They expanded the fur trade, founded banks, built the railroads and left their mark on the city architecturally in the form of stone and brick buildings. The late 20th century saw the "reconquest" of the city by the Québécois, and its face is now resolutely French.

Today, Montréal's economy is vibrant, with a strong high-tech orientation and a major port despite its location a thousand miles from the open ocean. The downtown area is flourishing, with the construction of some magnificent buildings, all interconnected by the passageways and plazas of the Underground City, born of Montréal's long, cold winter, which has an average snowfall of 3m (nearly 10ft), more than any other major city on Earth.

www.tourisme-montreal.org

✚ 9D

Centre Infotouriste

✉ 1255 rue Peel, Suite 100, Montréal, Québec, H3B 1N1 ☎ 514/873-2015; 877/266-5687 (toll free) 🕓 Jun–early Sep daily 7am–8pm; May and early Sep–Oct daily 7:30–6; Nov–Apr daily 9–6 🚇 Peel

ℹ 174 rue Notre-Dame Est ☎ 514/873-2015; 877/266-5687 (toll free) 🕓 Daily 9–5 (to 7pm late Jun–early Oct)

Basilique Notre-Dame de Montréal (Notre-Dame Basilica)

Built in 1923–29 the twin towers of Montréal's most famous Catholic church rise up over 69m (226ft) on the south side of place d'Armes.

The extraordinary interior of the church was the masterpiece of Victor Bourgeau, a local architect. It is handcarved in wood, mainly red pine, and decorated with 22-carat gold. Above the main altar, the reredos features scenes of sacrifice from the Bible sculpted in white pine. Don't miss the Chapelle du Sacre Coeur (Sacred Heart Chapel), rebuilt in 1982 after a fire, which is dominated by a 15m-high (50ft) bronze depicting humanity's journey through life towards heaven, the work of Charles Daudelin.

www.basiliquenddm.org

✠ *Montréal 6c* ✉ 110 rue Notre-Dame Ouest ☎ 514/842-2925; 866/842-2925 (toll free) 🕐 Daily ✋ Moderate (no charge for attending Mass) 🍴 Restaurants nearby ($–$$$) 🚇 Place d'Armes ❓ Guided tours

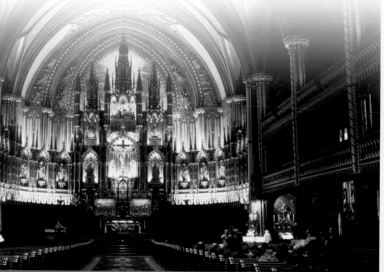

Biodôme

Within the former Olympic cycling stadium, four climate-controlled ecosystems have been created with real plantlife and animals. The areas represent a tropical forest, the Laurentian Forest, the underwater world of the St. Lawrence River, and polar regions. The many highlights include the penguins in the Polar World and taking refuge in the "tropics" on a winter's day.

www.biodome.qc.ca

➕ *Montréal 2f (off map)* ✉ 4777 avenue Pierre-de-Coubertin ☎ 514/868-3000 🕐 Daily 9–5 (to 6pm in summer). Closed Mon mid-Sep to Feb ✋ Expensive 🍴 Restaurants and cafés on site ($–$$) 🚇 Viau

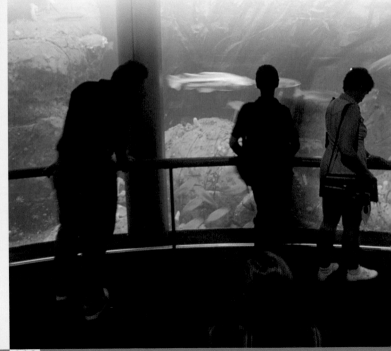

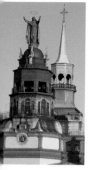

Cathédrale Anglicane de Christ Church
(Christ Church Cathedral)

Squeezed in between towering office blocks and a shopping center, this Anglican cathedral (built between 1856 and 1859) is a fine example of neo-Gothic architecture. It has a flamboyant triple portico on rue Ste-Catherine decorated with gables, gargoyles and grotesques, and a courtyard cloister at the back. Inside, walk up the nave below Gothic arches into the chancel, which has a copy of Leonardo da Vinci's *Last Supper*. Just above the pulpit, note the cross created from nails collected in the ruins of England's Coventry Cathedral after it was bombed in 1940.

www.montreal.anglican.org/cathedral

✚ *Montréal 2c* ✉ 635 rue Ste-Catherine Ouest ☎ 514/843-6577 ◷ Daily 🖐 Free 🍴 Restaurant in shopping mall beneath cathedral ($) 🚇 McGill ❓ Lunchtime concerts

Chapelle Notre-Dame-de-Bonsecours
(Chapel of Notre-Dame-de-Bonsecours)

This waterfront church was adopted by 19th-century sailors as their special church and a large statue of the Virgin with arms outstretched faces the river outside. Within the church, don't miss the grisaille frescoes, painted onto the wooden vault by François-Édouard Meloche in 1886. They recount scenes in the life of the Virgin and are executed in a *trompe l'oeil* style. The adjoining museum is devoted to Marguerite Bourgeoys, who settled in Montréal in 1653, built the original chapel on this site, and was canonized in 1982. There is a magnificent view from the tower.

www.marguerite-bourgeoys.com

✚ *Montréal 8f* ✉ 400 rue St-Paul Est ☎ 514/282-8670 ◷ May–Oct Tue–Sun 10–5:30; Nov to mid-Jan and Mar–Apr Tue–Sun 11–3:30; closed mid-Jan to Feb 🖐 Free. Museum: moderate 🍴 Restaurants nearby ($–$$$) 🚇 Champ-de-Mars ❓ Summer theatrical presentations; winter concerts

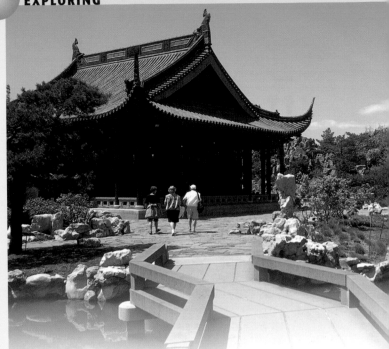

Jardin Botanique de Montréal (Montréal Botanical Gardens)

These splendid gardens extend over 73ha (180 acres). They consist of nearly 30 thematic gardens and 10 greenhouses with more than 22,000 different species from around the world. The Chinese Garden includes a number of pagodas set around a lake. The First Nations Garden has winding paths, trees and a lake populated with wildfowl. In summer, the gardens of annuals and perennials, and the rose garden, are glorious. The conservatories feature magnificent orchids, tropical plants, ferns and bonsai.

www.ville.montreal.qc.ca/jardin

✚ *Montréal 2f (off map)* ✉ 4101 rue Sherbrooke Est ☎ 514/872-1400
🕐 Daily 9–5 (to 6pm mid-May to early Sep; 9pm early Sep–Oct). Closed Mon early Jan to mid-May 🖑 Expensive May–Oct; moderate rest of year. Parking charge 🍴 Cafeteria ($) 🚇 Pie IX, Viau ❓ Guided tours; balade (small train) tour (free). Horticultural gift store

L'Oratoire St-Joseph (St. Joseph's Oratory)

Set on the north slope of Mont-Royal is the Roman Catholic shrine of L'Oratoire St-Joseph, whose huge dome is visible from all over the city. Founded in 1904, it is visited by millions every year and recent improvements to the site have enhanced access and facilities.

✚ *Montréal 1e (off map)* ✉ 3800 Chemin Queen-Mary ☎ 514/733-8211; 877/672-8647 (toll free); www.saint-joseph.org 🕐 Daily 🍴 Cafeteria ($) 🚇 Côte-des-Neiges ❓ Religious gift store

Mont-Royal

Best places to see, ➤ 42–43.

Musée d'Archéologie et d'Histoire de Montréal (Pointe-à-Callière Museum of Archeology and History)

Set on the point of land in Old Montréal where the city started life in 1642, this is an intriguing museum in a striking modern building. A short multimedia presentation provides an introduction to the history of the site. Then you can proceed down to an archeological crypt to inspect remains of the old city walls and buildings with

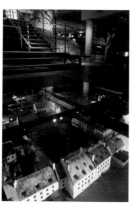

English- or French-speaking laser holograms acting as residents. Climb the stairs into the old Customs House for more exhibitions, or take the elevator up the tower for great views over the river.

www.pacmuseum.qc.ca

✚ *Montréal 7c* ✉ 350 place Royale ☎ 514/872-9150 🕐 Late Jun–Aug Mon–Fri 10–6, Sat–Sun 11–6; Sep–late Jun Tue–Fri 10–5, Sat–Sun 11–5 🖐 Expensive 🍴 Restaurant l'Arrivage ($$) 🚇 Place d'Armes ❓ Boutique with gifts and books at 150 rue St-Paul, Tue–Sun 11–6 (also Mon in summer)

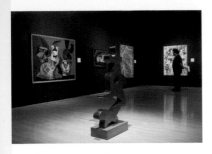

Musée d'Art Contemporain (Museum of Contemporary Art)

Montréal's contemporary art museum is part of the performing arts complex at Place des Arts (➤ 148), which also includes theaters and a concert hall. The museum building is recognizable by the pair of giant lips on its roof, called La Voie lactée (The Milky Way), an artwork by Geneviève Cadieux. This was the first museum in Canada devoted solely to contemporary art, and its approach remains innovative.

www.macm.org

✚ *Montréal 3e* ✉ 185 rue Ste-Catherine Ouest ☎ 514/847-622
🕓 Tue–Sun 11–6 (to 9pm Wed); also Mon late Jun–early Sep ✋ Moderate (free Wed 6–9pm) 🍴 Restaurant La Rotonde ($$$), café ($) 🚇 Place-des-Arts
🚌 15, 55, 80, 129, 535 ❓ Art bookstore and gift store

Musée des Beaux-Arts de Montréal (Montréal Museum of Fine Arts)

Featuring an encyclopedic collection of art dating from antiquity to contemporary times the musuem is spilt over two sites. On the north side of Sherbrooke Street, a Beaux-Arts building of 1912, houses the Canadian Collection, including some splendid Inuit works. Across the street is Moshe Safdie's 1991 pavilion, which hosts the galleries of European and contemporary art, as well as temporary exhibitions. Connecting the two are vast underground vaults lined with works of ancient civilizations (China, Japan and the Middle East), and African and pre-Columbian art.

www.mmfa.qc.ca

✚ *Montréal 1d (off map)* ✉ 1379 and 1380 rue Sherbrooke Ouest
☎ 514/285-2000; 800/899-6873 (toll free) 🕓 Tue 11–5, Wed–Fri 11–9, Sat–Sun 10–5 ✋ Permanent collection: free. Temporary exhibits: expensive
🍴 Restaurant ($$$), cafeteria ($) 🚇 Guy-Concordia 🚌 Bus 24

Parc Jean-Drapeau (Jean-Drapeau Park)

This park is composed of two islands and has a superb location in the middle of the St. Lawrence River that offers unparalleled views of the city. Together, Île Ste-Hélène and Île Notre-Dame provided the site for the 1967 World's Fair (Expo 67). Two of the former pavilions remain; one houses the Montréal Casino; the other, the Biosphère, an environmental museum. La Ronde amusement park (► 147) and the Stewart Museum are also located here.

www.parcjeandrapeau.com

✠ *Montréal 8f (off map)* ✉ 1 circuit Gilles-Villeneuve ☎ 514/872-6120 🕐 Daily 6am–midnight 🚇 Jean-Drapeau 🚌 Bus 169 access to islands, 167 on islands ⛴ Ferry from Jacques Cartier Pier, Vieux-Port late Jun–early Sep

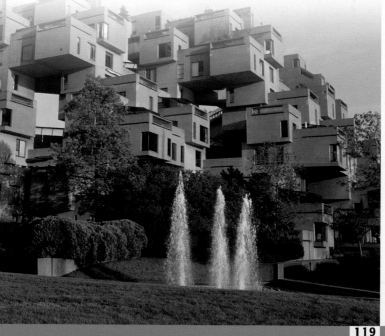

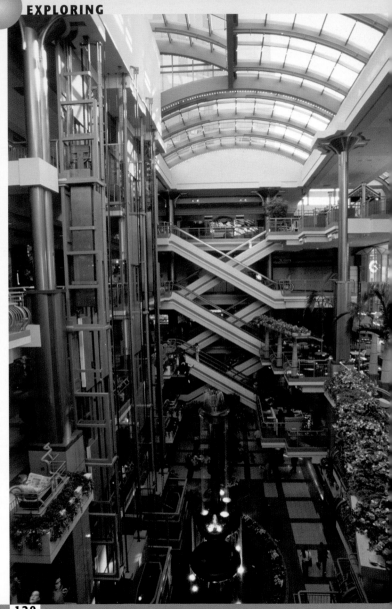

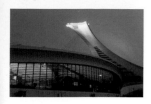

Parc Olympique (Olympic Park)

Site of the summer Olympic games of 1976, Olympic Park is dominated by a huge elliptical stadium that sports a leaning tower and strange roof. Controversial because of its cost, it is nonetheless a remarkable building and the view of the city from the top of the tower is spectacular. It rises to 175m (574ft) at an angle of 45 degrees, and ascent is via an external funicular that offers an exhilarating ride. Beside the stadium stands the Biodôme, which was used for the cycling events of the Olympic games (➤ 114).

www.rio.gouv.qc.ca

✚ *Montréal 2f (off map)* ✉ 4141 avenue Pierre-de-Coubertin ☎ 514/252-4141 🕐 Daily 9–5 (to 7pm mid-Jun to early Sep 🖐 Guided tours: moderate. Ascent of tower: expensive 🍴 Café 🚇 Pie IX, Viau ❓ Ball games and other sports events; trade shows

Underground City (Reseau Pietonnier Souterraine)

Montréalers have learned to cope with their harsh winters by developing a weatherproof system in downtown that gives priority to pedestrians. This network of passageways, atriums and wide open spaces, extends for more than 33km (20 miles) and connects more than 60 buildings, 40 entertainment venues and eight métro stations, is known as the Underground City, although not all of it is strictly underground. It all started with place Ville-Marie, the huge cruciform tower designed by I.M.Pei in 1962. Highlights include Le Complexe Les Ailes; Promenades Cathèdrale, an architecturally impressive complex below Christ Church Cathedral (➤ 115); Cours Mont-Royal complex, with its enclosed courtyards; the tallest building in the city, 1000 de la Gauchetière, with a spectacular indoor skating rink; and the high, light and luminous Centre de Commerce Mondial de Montréal.

✚ *Montréal 6d (Ville-Marie)*. Additional entrances across the city ❓ For details and maps, contact Centre Infotouriste: 1255 rue Peel, Suite 100 Montréal, Québec, H3B 4V4 ☎ 514/873-2015; 877/266-5687 (toll free)

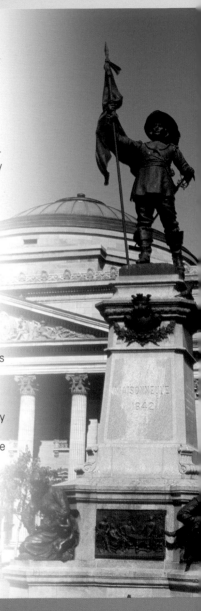

Vieux-Montréal (Old Montréal)

Close to the river, Old Montréal is a district of narrow, cobblestoned streets and old houses. It is the original French city, now a picturesque area that you can visit either by horse-drawn carriage or on foot. Don't miss place Jacques Cartier, with its outdoor cafés, street performers and flower vendors. At the north end of the square stands Montréal's magnificent Hôtel de Ville (City Hall), built in the French Second Empire style. Across the street is the venerable Château Ramezay, built in 1705 and today housing a local history museum. Rue St-Paul is the main thoroughfare, lined by boutiques, art galleries and restaurants in fine old buildings. The most prominent is the splendid, domed Marché Bonsecours, now full of high-quality craft retailers. Finally, don't miss place d'Armes, and the Notre-Dame Basilica (➤ 113).

www.vieux.montreal.qc.ca

✚ Montréal 7c

ℹ Centre Infotouriste (Vieux-Montréal): 174 rue Notre-Dame Est (on corner of place Jacques Cartier) ☎ 514/873-2015

🍴 Restaurants ($–$$$) 🚇 Champ-de-Mars, place d'Armes, Square Victoria

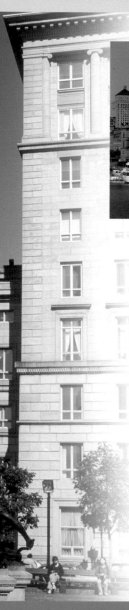

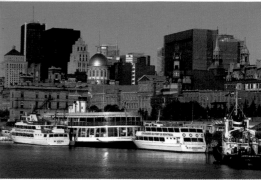

Vieux-Port (Old Port)

The Old Port is the name given to the area beside the St. Lawrence River south of rue de la Commune, which today forms an attractive linear waterfront park with great views of the city and river. Exhibitions, activities and festivals are held here throughout the year, and there is also the Centre des Sciences de Montréal (Montréal Science Centre; ➤ 67) to visit. The 45m (145ft) **Tour de l'Horloge** (Clock Tower), beside the river, can be climbed (192 steps) for a splendid view of the city. A variety of boat trips are on offer, including jet-boat rides over the Lachine Rapids.

www.quaysoftheoldport.com

✚ *Montréal 8d* ✉ 333 rue de la Commune Ouest, Montréal, Québec, H2Y 2E2 ☎ 514/496-7678; 800/971-7678 (toll free) 🍴 Cafés ($) 🚇 Champ-de-Mars, place d'Armes, Square Victoria

Tour de l'Horloge

✉ quai de l'Horloge, Vieux-Port de Montréal ☎ 514/496-7678; 800/971-7678 (toll free) 🕐 Late May–early Oct daily ✋ Free

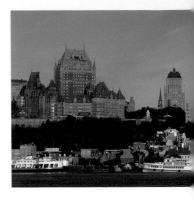

QUÉBEC CITY

Citadel, seaport and provincial capital, Canada's oldest city is built on a rock above the St. Lawrence. It has a distinct European flavor, with impressive fortifications and narrow cobblestoned streets lined with gray-stone buildings. True to its claim as the birthplace of French culture in North America, Québec City offers excellent restaurants, lively cafés and a vibrant nightlife.

In 1608, Samuel de Champlain built a trading settlement at the point "where the river narrows" (the meaning of the word Québec). Over the next 150 years, his settlement grew in size and importance to become the center of all activities in New France, an empire that stretched through the Great Lakes and south to the Gulf of Mexico. In 1759, a British fleet arrived under the command of James Wolfe and scaled the great rock face that provided Québec with its natural defense. The ensuing battle on the Plains of Abraham was won by the British, deciding the fate not only of the city but of the whole continent.

Today, it is a joy to explore Québec City's Haute-Ville, at the top of the cliff, and the Basse-Ville, below it at the foot. The steep cliffs are still impressive despite the construction of port facilities at their base, and the former battlefield is now a magnificent park covering 100ha (250 acres). In 1985, the combination of fortified site and French culture gave Québec a place on UNESCO's World Heritage List, one of only two Canadian cities to receive this honor (the other is Old Town Lunenburg ➤ 99).

www.quebecregion.com

✚ 10E

ℹ 12 rue Ste-Anne, Québec G1R 3X2 ☎ 418/649-2608; 877/266-5687 (toll free)

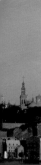

Cathédrale Notre-Dame de Québec (Notre-Dame Cathedral)
The Roman Catholic Cathedral of Notre-Dame has a rather undistinguished neoclassical facade that belies the opulence of the interior with its gold decoration. Over the altar, a vast wooden canopy is finished in gold, as are the pulpit and the bishop's throne. On the right side, a funeral chapel honors Monsignor de Laval, the first bishop of Québec; a map of his diocese – which extended over half the continent – is etched on the floor.
This is the third cathedral on this site. The first was destroyed by British bombardments in 1759, while the second burnt down in 1922. The present cathedral stands on the same foundations and was rebuilt using the original plans.
www.patrimoine-religieux.com

✉ 16 rue de Buade ☎ 418/692-2533 🕐 Daily from 7:30 (8:30 Sun). Closes at 4, 5 or 6pm depending on season 🖐 Inexpensive ❓ Guided tours

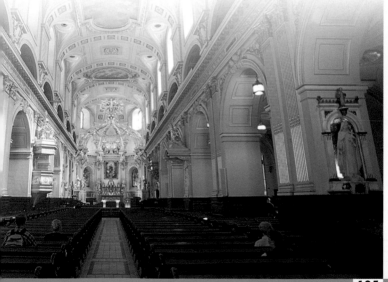

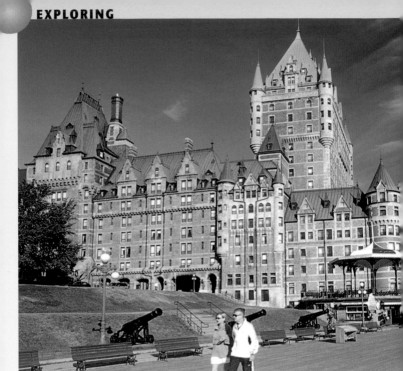

Château Frontenac

Inextricably linked with the image of the city, this striking and
famous hotel is named after a French governor, the Comte de
Frontenac. It towers flamboyantly above its surroundings, a
magnificent structure of turrets and copper roofs. The original hotel
was built by Bruce Price for the Canadian Pacific Railway in 1893,
and its architecture gave rise to the term "château style." Even if
you are not staying here, step inside to see the interior. During
World War II, the hotel hosted the Québec Conferences, when the
Normandy landings were planned by Franklin D. Roosevelt and
Winston Churchill.

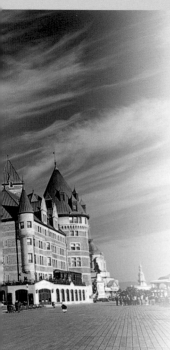

www.fairmont.com/frontenac
✉ 1 rue des Carrières ☎ 418/692-3861
🍴 Several restaurants and cafés in hotel
($–$$$) ❓ Guided tours (expensive and
popular); reservations (☎ 418/691-2166;
www.tourschateau.ca)

Citadelle (Québec Citadel)

This vast four-pointed polygon extends
over 15ha (37 acres) and remains an
active military base, home to the Royal
22e Régiment. It took the British more
than 30 years (1820–50) to complete
the vast array of earthworks and
bastions that make up the fort,
following a design by the French military
architect Vauban.

To visit the Citadel, you must join a
guided tour. Buildings bearing the
names of the various campaigns of the
Royal 22e Régiment (Vimy, the Somme
and so on) surround a huge parade
ground where military ceremonies take
place. Located in a powder magazine dating from 1750 is a
museum presenting military insignia, weapons, uniforms and an
excellent diorama showing the various battles fought at Québec.

From the Citadel, an entire network of walls and gates encircles
the old part of the city, stretching a total of 4.6km (2.8 miles).
www.lacitadelle.qc.ca
✉ Côte de la Citadelle ☎ 418/694-2815 🕐 Guided tours only; Apr daily
10–4; May–Jun daily 9–5; Jul–early Sep daily 9–6; Sep daily 9–4; Oct daily
10–3; Nov–Apr one tour daily 1:30pm. Changing of the Guard late Jun–early
Sep daily at 10am. Retreat ceremony early Jul–early Sep Fri 7pm
✋ Moderate

Holy Trinity Cathedral (Cathédrale de la Ste-Trinité)

Consecrated in 1804, this wood-framed Georgian church was the first Anglican cathedral to be built outside the British Isles. Modeled on the church of St. Martin-in-the-Fields in central London, it was paid for by King George III and still boasts a royal pew reserved for the sovereign. The light and spacious interior has box pews made of oak transported from England's royal forests. There is an impressive collection of stained glass: In the chancel, the triptych window portrays the Ascension, beside scenes of the Transfiguration and the Baptism. In the summer months, the cathedral courtyard is home to stalls selling local crafts.

http://209.160.3.218/

✉ 31 rue des Jardins ☎ 418/692-2193 ⊕ Mid-May to mid-Oct daily; mid-Oct to Apr Sun morning; open for services ♿ Free 🍴 Nearby ($–$$) ❓ Guided tours

Musée de la Civilisation (Museum of Civilization)

Inaugurated in 1988 and designed by architect Moshe Safdie, this building is a splendid example of how modern architecture can be integrated into the old city – incorporated within its walls is a four-story stone house, the Maison Estèbe, dating from 1751. Excavations carried out during construction unearthed many treasures. The museum is devoted to civilization in the broadest sense of the word, and the exhibitions (which change regularly) may feature life in any part of the world at any time. Among its permanent collection, there are fine examples of Québécois furniture, sculpture and crafts, as well as important First Nations artifacts.

www.mcq.org

✉ 85 rue Dalhousie ☎ 418/643-2158; 866/710-8031 (toll free) ⊕ Late Jun–early Sep daily 9–7; Tue–Sun 10–5, rest of year ♿ Moderate; free Tue, Nov–May and Sat 10–noon Jan–Feb 🍴 Cafeteria ($) 🚌 1 ❓ Gift store in Maison Estèbe

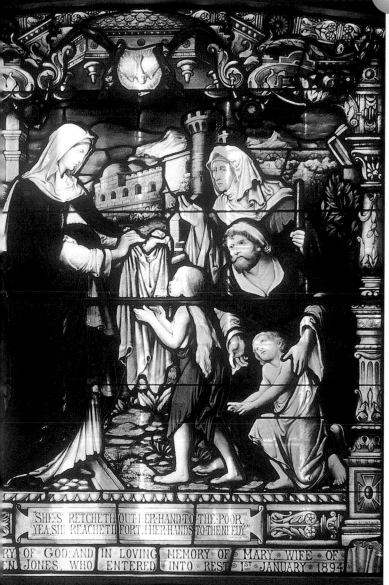

"SHE STRETCHETH OUT HER HAND TO THE POOR,
YEA SHE REACHETH FORTH HER HANDS TO THE NEEDY."

RY OF GOD AND IN LOVING MEMORY OF MARY WIFE OF
N JONES WHO ENTERED INTO REST 1ST JANUARY 1894

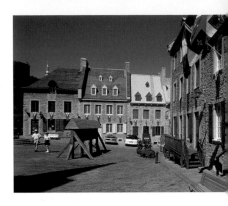

Place Royale

This picturesque square is in the center of the Basse-Ville (Lower Town) on the site where Samuel de Champlain built his first settlement in 1608. Today, it is lined with tall stone houses of French Regime style, with steeply pitched roofs and high chimneys (note the ladders on the roofs to enable people to climb up and sweep the chimneys). These houses were actually all rebuilt in the 1970s so that the square could take on the look it had at the time of the conquest, before it was blasted to bits by British mortar fire. A bust of King Louis XIV graces the center of the square, a copy of the original erected in 1686 that gave place Royale its name. On the west side stands the little church of Notre-Dame-des-Victoires with its distinctive steeple.

The narrow pedestrian streets around place Royale are perfect for exploration on foot. There are a number of craft stores along rue Petit-Champlain, antiques shops on rue St-Paul, and souvenir outlets just about everywhere.

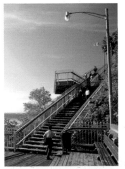

🍴 Restaurants/cafés ($–$$$) ❓ Access from Upper Town by funicular (inexpensive), or by descending the "Breakneck Steps" on foot

Promenade des Gouverneurs

Best places to see, ➤ 52–53.

Terrasse Dufferin

Best places to see, ➤ 52–53.

More to see in Québec Province

CANADIAN MUSEUM OF CIVILIZATION, GATINEAU

Best places to see, ➤ 36–37.

CHARLEVOIX COAST

On the north shore of the St. Lawrence River east of Québec City is the Charlevoix coast, where mountains sweep down to the water's edge and villages nestle in the valleys. There are ever-changing views of the river and shore, as well as possibilities for whale-watching (➤ 54–55). In 1989, the Charlevoix was named a UNESCO World Biosphere Reserve for its unique beauty.

The mountainous landscape of Charlevoix was created about 350 million years ago when a gigantic meteorite hit the Earth, making a crater that stretches some 56km (35 miles). Highlights of the region include Baie-St-Paul, whose beautiful location has long been a magnet for artists, and the rural charm of Île-aux-Coudres.

www.tourisme-charlevoix.com

✚ 10E ℹ Association touristique régionale de Charlevoix: 495 boulevard de Comporté, La Malbaie, Québec, G5A 3G3 ☎ 418/665-4454; 800/667-2276 (toll free) ❓ Ferry from St-Joseph-de-la-Rive to Île-aux-Coudres daily (free; ☎ 418/643-7308; www.traversiers.gouv.qc.ca)

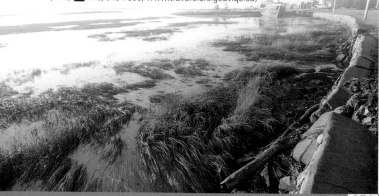

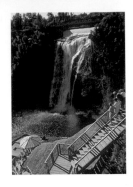

CHUTE MONTMORENCY (MONTMORENCY FALLS)

Near its junction with the St. Lawrence, the Montmorency River cascades over an 83m (272ft) cliff in an impressive waterfall. The spray it creates forms a great cone of ice up to 30m (100ft) high in the winter, known as the *pain de sucre* (sugarloaf). Tobogganing down the cone became a tradition in the 19th century and continues to this day. The falls and cliffs are illuminated at night.

Parc de la Chute Montmorency offers viewpoints at both the top and the bottom of the falls. At the top, a boardwalk takes you to a suspension bridge across the cataract that has spectacular views. At the bottom, you can walk right up to the whirlpool at the base of the falls. A cable car or steep staircase (487 steps) connects the upper and lower levels. The Manoir Montmorency at the top houses an interpretive center and restaurant.

www.sepaq.com

✚ 10E ✉ Parc de la Chute Montmorency, 2490 avenue Royal, Beauport, 12km (7.5 miles) east of Québec ☎ 418/663-3330
🕐 Upper Park: daily. Cable car and Lower Park: daily, Apr–Oct
✋ Parking fee (Apr–Oct): expensive. Cable car: expensive
🍴 Restaurant ($$) 🚌 Bus 50, 53 ❓ Craft store

EASTERN TOWNSHIPS (CANTONS DE L'EST)

Settled by Loyalists at the end of the 18th century, the Eastern Townships are a unique mixture of Anglo-Saxon ambience and French *joie de vivre*. They offer mountains rising nearly 1,000m (about 3,000ft) with a number of ski slopes, lakes perfect for boating and swimming, and quiet villages. Knowlton, near Brome Lake (famous for its

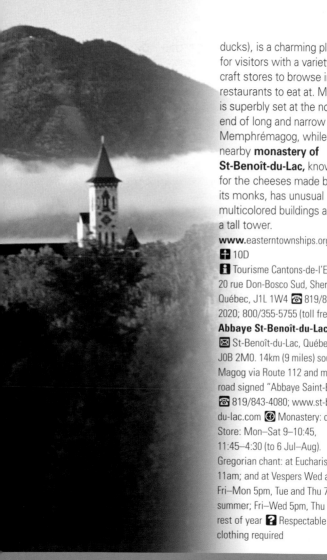

ducks), is a charming place for visitors with a variety of craft stores to browse in and restaurants to eat at. Magog is superbly set at the northern end of long and narrow Lake Memphrémagog, while the nearby **monastery of St-Benoît-du-Lac,** known for the cheeses made by its monks, has unusual multicolored buildings and a tall tower.

www.easterntownships.org

🗺 10D

🛈 Tourisme Cantons-de-l'Est: 20 rue Don-Bosco Sud, Sherbrooke, Québec, J1L 1W4 ☎ 819/820-2020; 800/355-5755 (toll free)

Abbaye St-Benoît-du-Lac

✉ St-Benoît-du-Lac, Québec, J0B 2M0. 14km (9 miles) south of Magog via Route 112 and minor road signed "Abbaye Saint-Benoît" ☎ 819/843-4080; www.st-benoit-du-lac.com 🎟 Monastery: daily. Store: Mon–Sat 9–10:45, 11:45–4:30 (to 6 Jul–Aug). Gregorian chant: at Eucharist daily 11am; and at Vespers Wed and Fri–Mon 5pm, Tue and Thu 7pm, summer; Fri–Wed 5pm, Thu 7pm, rest of year ❓ Respectable clothing required

ÎLE D'ANTICOSTI

Once a private hunting and fishing camp, the island of Anticosti in the Gulf of the St. Lawrence is today largely owned by the province of Québec and run as a nature reserve. Île d'Anticosti covers a massive 8,000sq km (3,000sq miles) and has much to offer nature lovers. There are more than 200 bird species (including bald eagles), a herd of white-tailed deer, impressive rock formations, caverns, waterfalls and the remains of about 200 shipwrecks off the rocky shores. Take the 3km (2-mile) hike up a canyon to see Vauréal Falls. Here, the river plunges 76m (249ft) into the steep-walled canyon.

www.sepaq.com

✚ 20K

ℹ️ Sépaq: Box 179, Port-Menier, Québec, G0G 2Y0 ☎ 418/535-0156

🚢 Relais Nordik (☎ 418/723-8787; www.groupedesgagnes.com)

✈️ Air Satellite (☎ 418/538-2332; www.airsatellite.com)

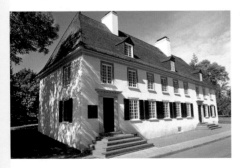

ÎLE D'ORLÉANS

The island of Orléans sits wedged like a giant cork in the St. Lawrence River as it widens beyond Québec City. In the early 17th century, French settlers began farming here and built the stone churches and Norman-style farmhouses that still grace its shores. In the summer months, the island becomes a vast open-air market, with fruit and vegetables on sale at roadside stands; it is especially famous for its strawberries. Route 368 makes a circular tour (about 70km/45 miles) of Île d'Orléans, giving some wonderful views of the tide-swept shores of the St. Lawrence and

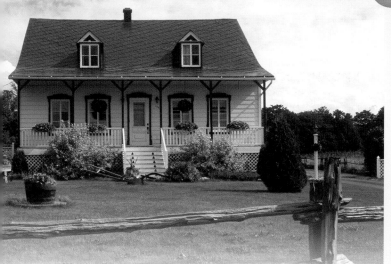

of Québec City. You will pass, and can visit, the **Manoir Mauvide-Genest,** a French manor house built in 1734 that has been splendidly restored. The small stone **church of St-Pierre,** built between 1717 and 1719, is no longer consecrated but it offers a veritable museum of religious art. The island also has some excellent restaurants.

www.iledorleans.com

✚ 10E 🛈 Chambre de commerce de l'Île d'Orléans: 490 côte du Pont, St-Pierre-de-l'Île d'Orléans, Québec, G04 4E0 ☎ 418/828-9411; 866/941-9411 (toll free)

Manoir Mauvide-Genest

✉ 1451 chemin Royal, St-Jean, Québec, G0A 3W0 ☎ 418/829-2630; www.manoirmauvidegenest.ca

🕙 Late Jun–Aug daily 10–5;
May–late Jun and Sep to mid-Oct
Sat–Sun 10–5 🖐 Moderate

Église St-Pierre

✉ 1249 chemin Royale, St-Pierre-de-l'Île d'Orléans, Québec, G0A 4E0

☎ 418/828-9824 🕙 May–Oct daily 🖐 Free

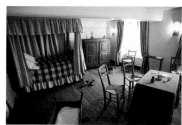

LAC ST-JEAN

Located north of Québec City, this large, saucer-shaped lake (1,350sq km/521sq miles) is the source of the Saguenay River (➤ 138). The land around is flat and fertile, and is particularly known for the wild blueberries *(bleuets)* that grow on its northern shore. In the water, a species of lake trout known as *ouananiche* flourishes, highly prized by sports fishermen. Lac St-Jean is renowned as the setting for *Maria Chapdelaine*, probably the most famous novel of French Canada ever written. In Péribonka, you can learn all about this love story at the **Musée Louis-Hémon**.

Set beside Ouiatchouan Falls, the former mill town of **Val-Jalbert** has been partially restored to recreate town-life in the 1920s. Don't miss climbing to the top of the falls (via 400 steps or a cable-car ride) for the view over the lake.

✚ 17H

Musée Louis-Hémon

✉ 700 route Maria Chapdelaine, Péribonka, Québec, G0W 2G0 ☎ 418/374-2177; www.museelh.ca 🕒 Jul–Aug daily 9–5; Sep–Jun Mon–Fri 9–4 ✋ Moderate

Village historique de Val-Jalbert

✉ Route 169, Chambord, Québec, G0W 1G0 ☎ 418/275-3132; 888/675-3132 (toll free); www.sepaq.com/ct/val/en/ 🕒 May–Oct daily ✋ Expensive

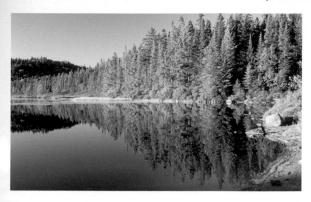

LES LAURENTIDES (LAURENTIANS)

When Montréalers talk of the "Laurentides," they are referring to the mountains just north of the city where ski centers and lakes abound. St-Sauveur-des-Monts is the region's oldest resort. At Ste-Agathe-des-Monts, you can take a **boat trip** around Lac-des-Sables (Sandy Lake). The **Tremblant complex** is an astounding place surrounded by wilderness; the buildings, with their colourful, steeply pitched roofs, house boutiques, bars, restaurants and accommodations of every type.

✚ 9D

Croisières Alouette

✉ Ste-Agathe-des-Monts,
Québec, J8C 3A3 ☎ 819/326-
3656; www.croisierealovette.com
🕐 Early Jun to late Oct daily
✋ Expensive

Tremblant complex

ℹ Information Centre, 48 chemin
de Brébeuf, Mont-Tremblant,
Québec, J8E 3Bl ☎ 819/425-
3300; 877/425-2434 (toll free);

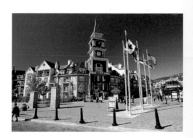

www.tourismemonttremblant.com 🕐 Daily 🍴 Restaurants/cafés ($$–$$$)

ROCHER PERCÉ, GASPÉSIE

Best places to see, ➤ 46-47.

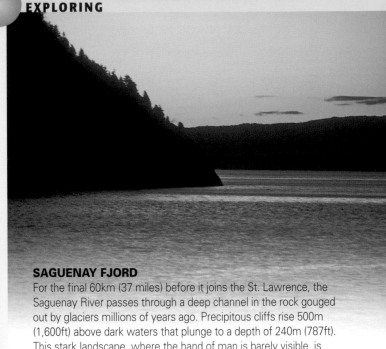

SAGUENAY FJORD

For the final 60km (37 miles) before it joins the St. Lawrence, the
Saguenay River passes through a deep channel in the rock gouged
out by glaciers millions of years ago. Precipitous cliffs rise 500m
(1,600ft) above dark waters that plunge to a depth of 240m (787ft).
This stark landscape, where the hand of man is barely visible, is
best appreciated by taking a **boat trip.** One highlight of the tour
is Cap Trinité, so named for the three ledges that punctuate its
face. On the first of these is a 9m-high (30ft) statue of the Virgin
carved in 1881, an awe-inspiring sight. There are also a few
viewpoints of the fjord from Routes 170 and 172, and at
Rivière-Éternité you can follow a steep trail up to the statue of
the Virgin (allow four hours return).

✚ 18H ℹ Fédération Touristique Régionale du Saguenay-Lac-St-Jean,
412 boulevard Saguenay Est, Bureau 100, Chicoutimi, Québec G7H 7Y8
☎ 418/543-9778; 877/253-8387 (toll-free);
www.tourismesaguenaylacsaintjean.qc.ca

Boat trips

Croisières La Marjolaine: Chicoutimi (☎ 418/543-7630; 800/363-7248
toll free); www.croisieremarjolaine.com

Rivière-Éternité walk

🕔 Mid-May to mid-Oct daily 🅿 Parking: expensive

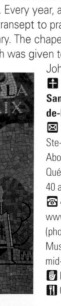

STE-ANNE-DE-BEAUPRÉ

This small community on the north shore of the St. Lawrence, has been a major place of pilgrimage for Roman Catholics since the early 1600s, when Breton sailors were brought safely to land here during a storm after praying to St. Anne. **Sanctuaire Ste-Anne-de-Beaupré,** the twin-spired basilica that dominates the site today, was inaugurated in 1934. Constructed of white granite in the form of a Latin cross, it has a magnificent interior with five naves, a barrel vault decorated with mosaics, and luminous stained-glass windows. Every year, a million or more pilgrims visit the basilica's north transept to pray before the statue of St. Anne holding the infant Mary. The chapel behind the statue contains a relic of the saint, which was given to the shrine by Pope John XXIII in 1960.

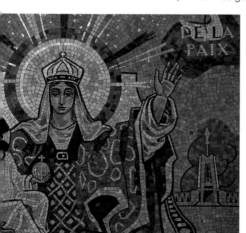

✚ 10E

Sanctuaire Ste-Anne-de-Beaupré

✉ 10018 avenue Royale, Ste-Anne-de-Beaupré. About 35km (22 miles) from Québec City via Highway 40 and Route 138

☎ 418/827-3781; www.ssadb.qc.ca 🕙 Daily (phone for times of Mass). Museum: Early Jun to mid-Oct daily 9–5

👖 Inexpensive

🍴 Cafeteria ($)

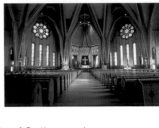

TADOUSSAC WHALE-WATCHING CRUISES

Best places to see, ➤ 54–55.

TROIS-RIVIÈRES

An industrial center known for its pulp and paper mills, Trois-Rivières is the third city of Québec province. As it joins the St. Lawrence here, the St. Maurice River branches around two islands – hence the name Trois-Rivières (Three Rivers). Close to the river, rue des Ursulines has some of the oldest-surviving buildings, the most striking of which is the Monastère des Ursulines (Ursuline Convent) of 1697. Nearby, a waterfront promenade offers views of the port and the Laviolette Bridge across the St. Lawrence. In neighboring Cap-de-la-Madeleine is

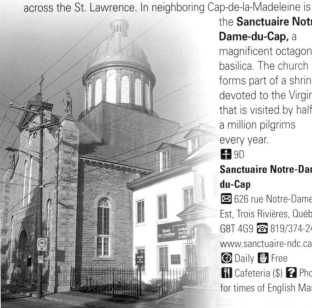

the **Sanctuaire Notre-Dame-du-Cap,** a magnificent octagonal basilica. The church forms part of a shrine devoted to the Virgin that is visited by half a million pilgrims every year.

✚ 9D

Sanctuaire Notre-Dame-du-Cap

✉ 626 rue Notre-Dame Est, Trois Rivières, Québec, G8T 4G9 ☎ 819/374-2441; www.sanctuaire-ndc.ca
🕐 Daily 🎫 Free
🍴 Cafeteria ($) ❓ Phone for times of English Masses

HOTELS

AYER'S CLIFF

▾▾▾ ▾▾▾ Auberge Ripplecove Inn ($$–$$$)

In lovely gardens overlooking Lake Massawippi in the Eastern Townships. Attractive hotel with an excellent restaurant, summer terrace and outdoor pool.

✉ 700 rue Ripplecove ☎ 819/838-4296; 800/668-4296 (toll free); www.ripplecove.com

BAIE-ST-PAUL

▾▾ ▾▾ Aux Portes du Soleil ($–$$)

In the heart of this lovely Charlevoix town, this is a stylish place to stay with good amenities, including free wireless internet, laundry and ski and snowshoe rental.

✉ 29 rue de la Lumière (Roue 362) ☎ 418/435-3540; www.auxportesdusoleil.com

MONTRÉAL

▾▾▾ Auberge de la Fontaine ($$$)

Pleasant, small hotel in a renovated Victorian house on Lafontaine Park in Montréal's east end. Generous Continental breakfast, and guests also have access to the kitchen to prepare their own meals.

✉ 1301 rue Rachel Est ☎ 514/597-0166; 800/597-0597 (toll free); www.aubergedelafontaine.com 🚇 Mont-Royal

▾▾▾ Château Versailles ($$$)

Luxury hotel in renovated former town houses with a modern extension across the street. Stylish bar and good restaurant.

✉ 1659 rue Sherbrooke Ouest ☎ 514/933-8111; 888/933-8111 (toll free); www.versailleshotels.com 🚇 Guy-Concordia

▾▾▾ ▾▾▾ Fairmont The Queen Elizabeth ($$$)

Grand dame of downtown accommodations, opened in 1958. Connected to Montréal's Underground City (➤ 121). John Lennon and Yoko Ono held their famous bed-in here. Indoor pool.

✉ 900 boulevard René-Lévesque Ouest ☎ 514/861-3511; 800/257-7544 (toll free); www.fairmont.com/queenelizabeth 🚇 Bonaventure, Peel, McGill

MONT-TREMBLANT
▽▽▽▽ Fairmont Tremblant ($$$)
Part of the enormous Tremblant resort complex, splendidly located with views of mountain and village. Rooms are standard – except for the views. Swimming pools and health club on site.

✉ 3045 chemin de la Chapelle ☎ 819/681-7000; 800/257-7544 (toll free); www.fairmont.com/tremblant

PERCÉ
▽▽▽▽ Le Mirage ($$–$$$)
Family-run hotel where every room has large windows and fabulous views of Percé's famous rock. Extensive grounds, tennis court and pool. Whale-watching boat trips can be arranged.

✉ 288 Route 132 Ouest ☎ 418/782-5151; 800/463-9011; www.hotellemirageperce.com 🅲 Closed mid-Oct to mid-May

QUÉBEC CITY
▽▽▽▽ Auberge Saint-Antoine ($$$)
In a once derelict warehouse in the Lower Town, this stylish boutique hotel has great originality and flair and includes themed suites.

✉ 8 rue St-Antoine ☎ 418/692-2211; 888/692-2211 (toll free); www.saint-antoine.com

▽▽▽▽ Fairmont Le Château Frontenac ($$$)
Dominates the Upper Town with its towers and turrets. Rooms are pleasant; those with any kind of view are expensive. Large swimming pool and spa; variety of restaurants.

✉ 1 rue des Carrières ☎ 418/692-3861; 800/257-7544 (toll free); www.fairmont.com/frontenac

▽▽ Gîte du Vieux-Bourg ($$)
This charming bed-and-breakfast, just a five-minute drive from downtown, occupies a historic stone house with a small art gallery and pool. Breakfast includes home-made bread and jam.

✉ 492 avenue Royale ☎ 418/661-0116; 866/661-0116 (toll free)

WAKEFIELD
◆◆◆ Wakefield Mill ($$)

Lovely inn in a 19th-century water mill on the La Pêche River north of Ottawa. Some rooms have exposed brick walls and hardwood floors, and some have views of the falls. Breakfast included.

✉ 60 Mill Road ☎ 819/459-1838; 888/567-1838 (toll free); www.wakefieldmill.com

RESTAURANTS

MONTRÉAL
◆◆ Alpenhaus ($$)

On the corner with busy rue Ste-Catherine. Swiss restaurant specializing in fondues, veal escalopes and entrecôte steaks.

✉ 1279 rue St-Marc ☎ 514/935-2285; www.restaurantalpenhaus.com
🕓 Mon–Wed 12–3pm, 5:30–10pm, Thu 12–10, Fri 12–10:30, Sat 4:30–10:30, Sun 5:30–10 🚇 Guy-Concordia

◆◆ Bar-B Barn ($)

A barn of a place with no frills, but the ribs are great and the chicken's not bad either.

✉ 1201 rue Guy ☎ 514/931-3811; www.barbbarn.ca 🚇 Guy-Concordia

◆◆ Café des Beaux-Arts ($$)

In the Montréal Museum of Fine Arts, this restaurant is as elegant as the surrounding art. Venison and duck are on the menu.

✉ 1384 rue Sherbrooke Ouest ☎ 514/843-3233; www.mmfa.qc.ca/services/cafe_des_beaux_arts 🕓 Tue–Sun 11:30–2:30; Wed 6–9
🚇 Guy-Concordia

◆◆ Delmo ($$)

Beautifully renovated bistro serving French classics like *moules marinère* and *bouillabaisse* and the occasional Canadian dish, such as *Bavette de bison*.

✉ 211 rue Notre-Dame Ouest ☎ 514/335-1869; www.delmo.ca
🕓 Mon–Tue 11–11, Wed–Sat 11am–midnight, Sun 5:30–11

▼▼▼ Gibby's ($$$)

In fine stone buildings in Old Montréal. First and foremost a steak house, though there is also plenty of fish on the menu.

✉ 298 place d'Youville ☎ 514/282-1837; www.gibbys.com ⊙ Sun–Fri from 5pm, Sat from 4:30pm Ⓜ Place Victoria

▼▼ House of Jazz/Maison de Jazz ($$)

This club has a long tradition of providing great ribs and the best jazz in the city.

✉ 2060 rue Aylmer ☎ 514/842-8656; www.houseofjazz.ca ⊙ Mon–Wed 11:30am–12:30am, Thu 11:30am–1:30am, Fri 11:30am–2:30am, Sat 6pm–2:30am, Sun 6pm–12:30am Ⓜ McGill, Place-des-Arts

▼▼▼ Milos ($$$)

Top-notch Greek restaurant with the freshest fish and vegetables in the city, flown in directly from Greece on occasion.

✉ 5357 avenue du Parc ☎ 514/272-3522; www.milos.ca ⊙ Mon–Fri 12–3, 5:30–late, Sat–Sun from 5:30pm 🚌 Bus 80 ❓ Valet parking

▼▼▼ Le Piment Rouge ($$$)

Sophisticated, elegant restaurant serving excellent, well-presented Szechuan shrimp, chicken, duck and beef dishes.

✉ Le Windsor, 1170 rue Peel ☎ 514/866-7816; www.lepimentrouge.ca ⊙ Mon–Thu 11:30–11, Fri 11:30am–midnight, Sat 12–12, Sun 12–11 Ⓜ Peel

▼▼ Reuben's Deli ($)

Famous for its 10-ounce smoked-meat sandwich, Reuben's also serves prime-aged steaks, chops, burgers, salads and desserts.

✉ 1116 rue Ste-Catherine Ouest ☎ 514/866-1029; www.reubensdeli.com ⊙ Daily 6:30am–2:30am

▼▼ Stash Café ($–$$)

In Old Montréal. Popular bistro-type restaurant serving Polish fare such as *pirogies*, cabbage rolls, sauerkraut stew and borscht.

✉ 200 rue St-Paul Ouest ☎ 514/845-6611; www.stashcafe.com ⊙ Daily 11:30–11:30 Ⓜ Place d'Armes

MONT-TREMBLANT
✇ Microbrasserie Le Diable ($)
Really bustles in the evening, especially popular with skiers.
Excellent beer brewed on the spot.
✉ 117 chemin Kandahar ☎ 819/681-4546 🕓 Daily 11:30am–3am

PERCÉ
✇✇✇ La Normandie Dining Room ($$–$$$)
Sensational location overlooking Rocher Percé. Seafood and fish
dishes with great originality and flair.
✉ 221 route 132 Ouest ☎ 418/782-2112; 800/463-0820 (toll free);
www.normandieperce.com 🕓 Dinner only. Closed Oct–early Jun

QUÉBEC CITY
✇✇ Aux Anciens Canadiens ($$)
Charming restaurant in a 17th-century house in the Upper Town.
Specializes in traditional Québec cuisine.
✉ 34 rue St-Louis ☎ 418/692-1627; www.auxancienscanadiens.qc.ca
🕓 Daily 12–9

✇✇ Au Petit Coin Breton ($$)
In the Upper Town of Old Québec. Nearly 80 varieties of crêpes.
✉ 1029 rue St-Jean ☎ 418/694-0758 🕓 Mon–Wed 11–2, 5–9, Thu–Fri
11–10, Sat 9am–10pm

✇✇✇ Charles-Baillairgé ($$$)
Classy, popular restaurant in the Clarendon Hotel in Upper Town.
Refined cuisine and piano chamber music.
✉ Hotel Clarendon, 57 rue Ste-Anne ☎ 418/692-2480; 888/222-3304;
www.dufour.ca 🕓 Mon–Fri 7–10:30am, 11:30–2, 6–9:30, Sat–Sun 7–10:30,
6–9:30

✇✇ Le Cochon Dingue ($$)
Café-bistro par excellence in Lower Town. Excellent *frites* (fries),
mussels and desserts.
✉ 46 boulevard Champlain ☎ 418/692-2013; www.cochondingue.com
🕓 Daily 7am–11pm

♦♦ ♦♦ Laurie Raphael ($$$)

In the Old Port area of Lower Town. International cuisine with a contemporary flavor. Reservations essential.

✉ 117 rue Dalhousie ☎ 418/692-4555; www.laurieraphael.com 🕘 Tue–Fri 11:30–2, 5:30–10, Sat 5:30–10. Closed Sun, Mon

SHOPPING

SHOPPING CENTERS AND MALLS
Complexe Desjardins

On east side of downtown linked to the Underground City. Has a vast central atrium. Good choice of fashion stores.

✉ 150 rue Ste-Catherine Ouest or 175 boulevard René-Lévesque Ouest, Montreal ☎ 514/281-1870; 514/845-4636 (info-line) 🚇 Place-des-Arts

Place Laurier

West of downtown. Largest mall in Québec, with 350 stores, including Zellers, The Bay, and Sears. Food court and restaurants.

✉ 2700 boulevard Laurier, Québec City ☎ 418/651-5000

MARKETS
Atwater Market

Popular daily market selling local produce, cheese, meat, fish and bread. Acres of flowers in the spring; fruit and vegetables all summer and maple products year-round. Café.

✉ 138 avenue Atwater, Montréal ☎ 514/937-7754; www.marchpublicsmtl.com 🚇 Lionel-Groulx

Québec Public Market

In the Old Port. Sells great cheese and bread, wonderful fruit in season, maple products and flowers.

✉ 160 quai St-Andre, Quebec City ☎ 418/692-2517

CRAFTS, ANTIQUES AND OTHER SPECIALTIES
Antiquités Hier pour Demain

Québec pine furniture, woodcarvings, folk art and old toys.

✉ 914 boulevard des Laurentides, Piedmont ☎ 450/227-4231
🕘 Closed Mon–Thu

Boutique Au Bon Secours

An artisan-owned craft store in a former pharmacy selling original work by local artists, notably sandstone bird sculptures.

✉ 150 route 138 Ouest, Percé ☎ 418/782-2011 🕐 Closed Nov–Apr

Galeries d'Art Inuit Brousseau et Brousseau

Next door to the Château Frontenac. Store and gallery devoted to the works of Canada's Inuit artists and sculptors.

✉ 35 rue St-Louis, Québec City ☎ 418/694-1828; www.sculpture.artinuit.ca

Henri Henri

The hat store to beat all hat stores. Great fur hats and classic headgear for men by names such as Biltmore and Stetson.

✉ 189 rue Ste-Catherine Est, Montréal ☎ 514/288-0109; 888/388-0109; www.henrihenri.ca 🚇 St-Laurent, Berri-UQAM

Ogilvy

In business since 1866. Home to 20 or more fashion franchises. Famous for its bagpiper, who parades through the store at noon.

✉ 1307 rue Ste-Catherine Ouest, Montréal ☎ 514/842-7711 🚇 Peel

ENTERTAINMENT

CHILDREN'S ENTERTAINMENT

Parc Omega

Drive-through enclosure where you can see buffalo, moose and bear in their natural habitats. On foot, you can explore the deer enclosure and otter pool. Restaurant.

✉ 323 North Road, Montebello ☎ 819/423-5487; www.parc-omega.com 🕐 Daily 9–6 (last admission 5pm). Closes one hour earlier Nov–May ✋ Expensive

La Ronde

Québec's biggest amusement park has more than 40 rides including Goliath, one of the fastest rollercoasters in North America.

✉ 22 Chemin Macdonald, Île Sainte-Hélène, Montréal (Québec) ☎ 514/397-7777; www.laronde.com 🕐 Late May–early Sep daily; Sep–Oct weekends ✋ Expensive 🚇 Jean-Drapeau 🚌 167, 169

THEATERS AND NIGHTCLUBS

Cabaret Mado

Renowned Montréal drag queen, Mado Lamotte, owns and runs this cabaret club in the Gay Village, featuring comedy shows, drag extravaganzas, dance nights and karaoke.

✉ 1115 rue Ste-Catherine Est, Montréal ☎ 514/525-7566; www.mado.qc.ca

Café Chaos

Long-established live music venue featuring emerging local bands, DJ theme nights and free Happy Hour acoustic shows.

✉ 2031 rue St-Denis ☎ 514/844-0738; www.cafechaos.qc.ca 🚇 Berri-UQAM or Sherbrooke

Comedyworks

On the second floor of Jimbo's Pub. Improv comedy during the week and big-name shows on weekends.

✉ 1238 rue Bishop, Montréal ☎ 514/398-9661; www.comedyworksmontreal.com 🚇 Guy-Concordia, Lucien L'Allier

House of Jazz/Masion de Jazz

See page 144.

Grand Théâtre du Québec

Home to the Opéra du Québec and the Québec Symphony Orchestra. Annual program of dance, music and French theater.

✉ 269 boulevard René-Lévesque Est, Québec City ☎ 418/643-8131; www.grandtheatre.qc.ca

Place des Arts

Montréal's major performing arts center, with a concert hall, four theaters, and the Museum of Contemporary Art. Classical music, opera, ballet and live theater year-round.

✉ 175 rue Ste-Catherine Ouest, Montréal ☎ 514/842-2112; 866/842-2112 (toll-free); www.pda.qc.ca 🚇 Place-des-Arts

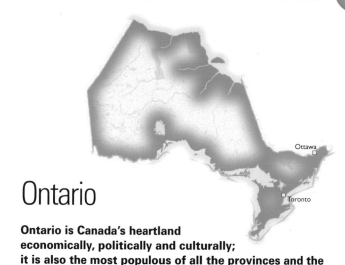

Ontario

**Ontario is Canada's heartland
economically, politically and culturally;
it is also the most populous of all the provinces and the
richest. The waters of four
of the five Great Lakes
wash its shores and it takes
its name from one of them.
In fact, the word Ontario
actually means "shining
waters," an apt description
of a province that includes
200,000sq km (70,000sq
miles) of lakes.**

The beauty of such natural regions as the Thousand Islands and
Georgian Bay is closely associated with water, and Ontario's major
cities are all located either beside a lake or next to a large river.
Thunder Bay lies on Lake Superior, Sault Ste. Marie is on the St.
Mary's River, Ottawa has an impressive site on the river of the
same name, and Toronto – the province's capital and Canada's
largest city and financial center – sits majestically on the northern
shore of Lake Ontario. Last but not least, the province boasts the
magnificent spectacle of Niagara Falls, one of the world's great
tourist attractions.

OTTAWA

As befits a nation's capital, Ottawa has its fair share of imposing architecture: The Parliament Buildings are a masterpiece of Gothic fantasy and some of the national museums are splendidly housed. But visitors tend to remember the beautiful drives by the river, the canal (which becomes a vast skating rink in the winter), the tulips in May and the stalls of fresh produce at the Byward Market.

Ottawa wasn't originally intended to be the capital. It started life as a raucous lumber town and was taken over by the military when the Rideau Canal was built in the 1820s. Queen Victoria considered both Montréal and York (now Toronto) too close to the U.S. border to be the new capital of her colony, so in 1857 she chose "Bytown" instead. This choice did not please everyone, and the city was soon nicknamed "Westminster in the Wilderness" by its detractors. The inhabitants, however,

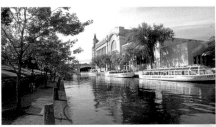

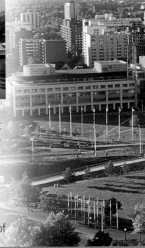

renamed their home after the river on which it stands. And since the Ottawa River marks the boundary between the provinces of Ontario and Québec, between English-speaking and French-speaking Canada, it did indeed prove to be a good choice.

Today, Ottawa is very much a city of government, and is not ruled by the temples of finance as are Toronto and Montréal. Instead, the highrise buildings contain government departments and some of the most expensive homes here are owned by civil servants. But Ottawa is not a contrived place created to impress people with the greatness of Canada. In many ways, it defies the image many people have of what a capital city ought to be. It is in the end quintessentially Canadian.

✚ 9D

National Capital Commission Infocentre

✉ 90 Wellington Street (opposite Parliament Buildings), Ottawa, Ontario, K1P 5A1 ☎ 613/239-5000; 800/465-1867 (toll free); www.canadascapital.gc.ca ⊕ Daily

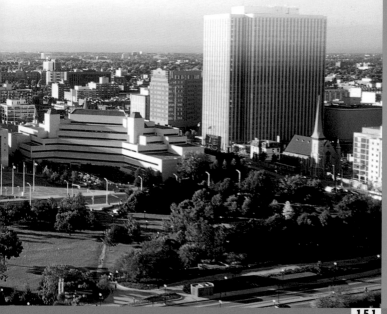

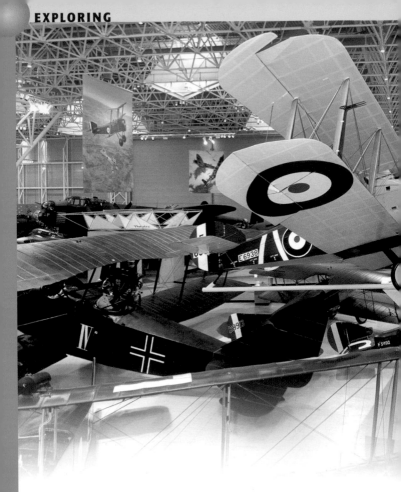

Canada Aviation Museum
Housed in a huge triangular hangar, the Canada Aviation Museum
is home to the most comprehensive collection of aircraft in Canada
which illustrate the story of aeronautical history. Many deem it to
be the most impressive collection of vintage aircraft in the world,
which is not too surprising when one considers how important
airplanes have been in opening up Canada.

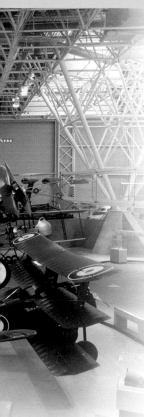

The Walkway of Time takes you on a journey through the different eras of aviation development. You can relive the adventures of Canada's bush pilots and see examples of the De Havilland Beaver (this plane was the prototype of a total of 1,600 that were built), and the Twin Otter, two of Canada's most important contributions to international aviation. You can even venture on a virtual-reality hang glider!

www.aviation.technomuses.ca

✉ 11 Aviation Parkway ☎ 613/993-2010; 800/463-2038 (toll free) ⏰ May–early Sep daily 9–5; early Sep–Apr Wed–Sun 10–5 🖐 Moderate; free 4–5pm. Parking: free 🍴 Café ($) ❓ Aeronautica gift shop

Canada Science and Technology Museum

This fascinating museum is devoted to the ingenuity of Canadian inventions, and every aspect of the scientific spectrum is featured – from the snowmobile to the Canadarm (part of the space shuttle). With its profusion of waterways, Canada was largely explored by canoe, and the museum has an excellent display detailing its development. The Locomotive Hall is another highlight, with an incredible display of huge and powerful locomotives. There's a splendid account of Canada in space, which features a popular simulator. In it you can "travel" to Mars to save a colony whose generator has been damaged by meteorites.

www.sciencetech.technomuses.ca

✉ 1867 St. Laurent Boulevard ☎ 613/991-3044; 866/442-4416 (toll free) ⏰ May–early Sep daily 9–5; early Sep–Apr Tue–Sun 9–5 🖐 Moderate; additional charge for the Simex Virtual Voyages™ Simulator

Canadian War Museum

From the early days of New France through two world wars to present-day peacekeeping duties for the United Nations, Canada has had an interesting military history. This is splendidly brought to life at the Canadian War Museum through the use of life-size dioramas and displays. Highlights include memorabilia from the Battle of Vimy Ridge in 1917, the D-Day landings of 1944 (including a Mercedes-Benz car used by Adolf Hitler), and Korea in the 1950s. A more modern acquisition is the Iltis jeep used by Canadian peacekeepers wounded in Bosnia.

www.civilization.ca

✉ 1 Vimy Place ☎ 819/776-8600; 800/555-5621 (toll free) 🕙 May to mid-Oct daily 9–6 (to 9pm Thu; also to 9pm Fri Jul–early Sep); mid-Oct to Apr Tue–Sun 9–5 (to 9pm Thu) 🖐 Moderate; free Thu 4–9, Jul 1 and Nov 11 🍴 The Mess ($), May to mid-Oct ❓ Gift store

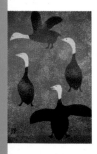

National Gallery of Canada

Masterpiece of architect Moshe Safdie, the National Gallery of Canada is a visually stunning building with a tower whose glittering prisms echo the Gothic turrets of the Parliamentary Library across the Rideau Canal. It occupies a splendid site in the heart of the city with wonderful views of the Canadian Parliament. Inside, the Great Hall has more splendid views, and the long, elegant galleries, courtyards and skylights diffuse natural light throughout the building.

The gallery is home to more than 1,500 works of Canadian art, from the religious works of New France to today's contemporary presentations. Don't miss the Rideau Chapel, which has a neo-Gothic fan-vaulted ceiling; the Croscup Room, with naive murals painted in Nova Scotia; and the rooms of Inuit art that are hidden away in the basement. The gallery also has an important European collection and hosts major temporary exhibitions.

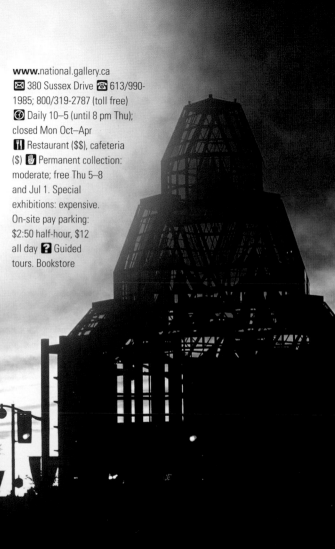

www.national.gallery.ca

✉ 380 Sussex Drive ☎ 613/990-1985; 800/319-2787 (toll free)

🕐 Daily 10–5 (until 8 pm Thu); closed Mon Oct–Apr

🍴 Restaurant ($$), cafeteria ($) ✋ Permanent collection: moderate; free Thu 5–8 and Jul 1. Special exhibitions: expensive. On-site pay parking: $2:50 half-hour, $12 all day ❓ Guided tours. Bookstore

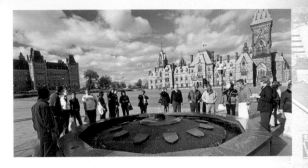

Parliament Hill

The three buildings of the Canadian Parliament stand on a high bluff above the Ottawa River and are commonly referred to as Parliament Hill. Neo-Gothic in their architectural inspiration, their copper roofs, carved stonework, turrets and towers are nothing if not picturesque. The East and West blocks (which house offices) date from the 1860s, while the Centre Block (which houses the House of Commons and the Senate) was rebuilt after a fire in 1916. At the center of the latter is the Peace Tower, 91m (300ft) high and added in 1927 as a monument to Canadians killed during World War I; it contains a carillon of 53 bells.

From Wellington Street, walk around the exterior of the buildings (you will pass the Info-Tent, where tours of the interior start in summer). There are wonderful views of the Ottawa River and Gatineau, Québec, as well as monuments to Canadian politicians. Overlooking the river is the Gothic structure that houses the Parliamentary Library, the only part of the Centre Block to survive the 1916 fire.

www.canadascapital.gc.ca

🕐 Daily 🛈 National Capital Commission Infocentre: 90 Wellington Street (opposite Parliament Buildings) ☎ 613/239-5000; 800/465-1867 (toll free) 🖐 Free ❓ Guided tours leave from Info-Tent. Mid-May to late Jun daily 9–5; late Jun–early Sep daily 9–8; from Visitor Welcome Centre in Centre Block rest of year. Changing of the Guard: late Jun–late Aug daily 10am. Sound and light shows: late Jun–late Aug daily ☎ 613/239-5000 for times and language ❓ Visitors have to go

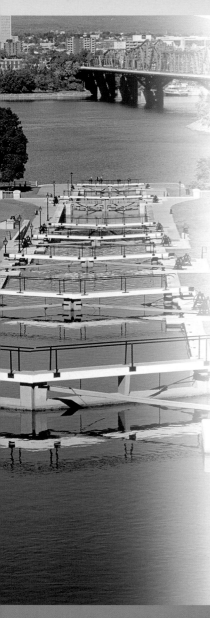

through a security check before
entering Parliament buildings

Rideau Canal and Locks
Today, this canal – built in the
1820s as a military route
between Ottawa and Kingston
(➤ 170) – forms an attractive
linear park as it cuts right
through the heart of the capital.
You can stroll or join the
joggers beside it, or take a boat
cruise along it. In the winter
months, it becomes a 7.8km-
long (4.8-mile) skating rink.
Between Parliament Hill and
the Château Laurier Hotel, the
canal descends to the Ottawa
River via a series of eight flight
locks. In the shadow of serious
parliamentary business, it's
diverting to watch the pleasure
craft cruising up and down.
www.canadascapital.gc.ca
ℹ National Capital Commission
Infocentre: 90 Wellington Street
(opposite Parliament Buildings)
☎ 613/239-5000; 800/465-1867
(toll free); 613/239-5234 (ice
conditions) ? Boat cruises
(expensive) run mid-May to mid-Oct
daily: Paul's Boat Lines Ltd
(☎ 613/225-6781; 613/235-8409;
www.paulsboatcruises.com)

TORONTO

Set on the north shore of Lake Ontario, and with a skyline dominated by the CN Tower, Toronto is an amazingly diverse city. It is a great North American metropolis, vastly wealthy and powerful in financial terms, with a population that is both eclectic and ethnically mixed. There are districts where you are transported to China, Korea or India; to Italy, Portugal or Greece; to Poland, Hungary or Ukraine; and to Chile, San Salvador or Jamaica.

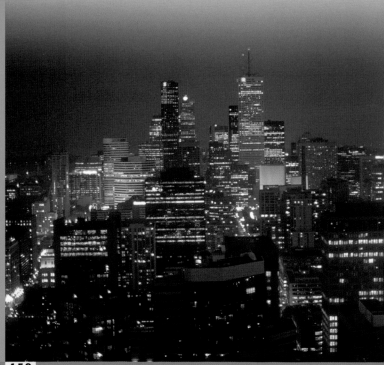

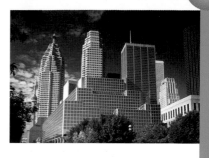

In 1793, Governor John Graves Simcoe decided to locate the new capital of Upper Canada on a swampy site north of Lake Ontario. He called it York after one of the sons of George III, but it was soon nicknamed "Muddy York" because of the state of its streets. In 1813, the Americans burned it to the ground, but it rose from the ashes to become, by the end of the 19th century, a bastion of Anglo-Saxon rectitude. By the 1920s, it was known as "Toronto the Good" and Prohibition reigned.

After World War II, the Ontario capital slowly started to blossom. Immigrants poured in from every corner of the world, providing a stimulating mix of social activities and making it one of the world's most ethnically varied cities. Gradually, Toronto took over from Montréal as Canada's economic heart. In the downtown area close to the lake, the country's great fiscal institutions have vied to build bigger and more impressively than one another. As a result, modern-day Toronto boasts an attractive skyline and some spectacular contemporary architecture. It offers a range of interesting attractions for the visitor, including some innovative cultural institutions housing collections to rival those of the world's greatest museums, again displaying some stunning modern architecture.

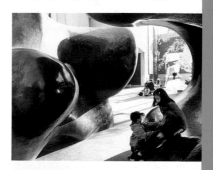

www.torontotourism.com

✚ 7B

ℹ️ 207 Queens Quay West, Toronto, Ontario, M5J 1A7

☎ 416/203-2600; 800/499-2514 (toll free) 🕐 Mon–Fri during business hours

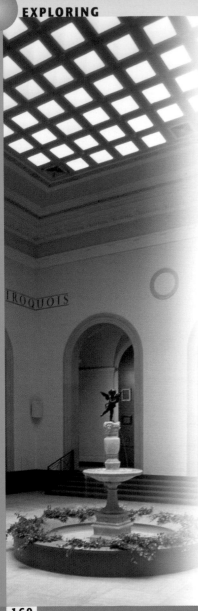

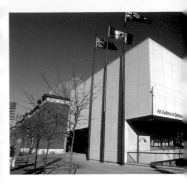

Art Gallery of Ontario

In November 2008 the expanded and transformed AGO reopened, marking the end of an ambitious and inspirational project that has added more than 9,000sq m (97,000sq ft) of gallery space and renovated some 17,600sq m (190,000sq ft) of the existing building, at a cost of $254 million. The stunning new building, by internationally acclaimed architect Frank Gehry, has vastly enhanced what was already one of the finest art galleries in the world, flooding the building with natural light and offering tantalizing glimpses of some of its treasures to passersby on the street.

The project was prompted by the gift of the

magnificent art collection of Ken Thomson, including important European masterpieces and pivotal works by leading Canadian artists. These works add to the gallery's already remarkable collections, which span all periods, genres and media.

The many highlights of the gallery include the Henry Moore Sculpture Centre, housing the world's largest public collection – some 900 pieces – of the works of the great British sculptor.

www.ago.net

✝ *Toronto 2d* ✉ 317 Dundas Street West ☎ 416/979-6648 🕓 Wed–Fri 12–9, Sat–Sun 10–5:30 ✋ Expensive; free Wed 6–9pm 🍴 Restaurant ($$), café ($) Ⓜ St. Patrick 🚌 Dundas streetcar 505 ❓ Gift and book store

CN Tower

Best places to see, ➤ 40–41.

Distillery District

In 2003 a lively new district burst onto the Toronto scene, a National Historic Site created out of the abandoned complex of the old Gooderham and Worts distillery. Established in the 1830s, the distillery was at one time producing more than 2 million gallons of whiskey a year, but the business declined during the 20th century and eventually closed in 1990.

Now, the 44 splendidly preserved Victorian industrial buildings, linked by cobblestoned streets and covering more than 5 hectares (13 acres), are home to artists' studios and galleries, upscale boutiques, theaters, restaurants, cafés and cultural venues, including the Young Centre for the Peforming Arts. There's a farmers' market every Sunday and a full program of events throughout the year. In common with the rest of Toronto (aka "Hollywood North") the district is a popular filming location.

www.thedistillerydistrict.com

✝ *Toronto 4b (off map)* ✉ Mill Street ☎ 416/364-1177 🍴 Restaurants and cafés on site ($–$$$) Ⓜ Castle Frank, then bus 65A south, or Union Station then bus 🚌 65A, 72, 172; King streetcar 504 to Parliament Street

Harbourfront Centre

Over the past 30 years, the city's industrial docklands have been renovated to create a recreational and cultural attraction that draws thousands of visitors every year. Part of Harbourfront's popularity lies in the infinite variety of the activites it offers. Some go there just to wander along the waterfront and to admire the views; others go to shop at the chic stores of Queens Quay Terminal, or to eat at one of the restaurants there. Some head for York Quay Terminal, with studios housing craftspeople at work; still others take part in one of the many cultural events held here.

www.harbourfrontcentre.com

✚ *Toronto 3a* ✉ South of Queens Quay West between York Street and Spadina Avenue ☎ 416/973-4000 ⏰ Daily 10am–11pm (to 9pm Sun) ♿ Free. Parking: expensive 🍴 Restaurants and cafés ($–$$$) Ⓢ Union or Spadina, then streetcar 🚌 Harbourfront streetcar 509, 510

Kensington Market

The warren of small streets around Kensington Avenue offers an amazing potpourri of businesses. Houses have been converted into shops, and casual restaurants and stores spill out onto the street. Chilean butchers, Italian fishmongers and Portuguese spice merchants stand cheek by jowl with Jamaican fast-food stands and Laotian eateries. You can buy spices, unusual vegetables, fish, cheeses and breads. With its incredible cacophony of sounds it may

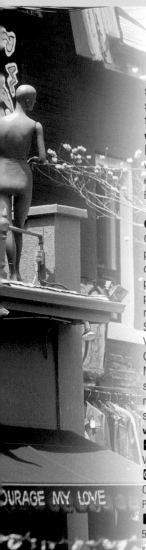

seem chaotic, but if you want to buy carpets, secondhand furniture or vintage clothing, there's no place like it.

www.kensington-market.ca

✚ *Toronto 1d* ✉ North of Dundas Street West and west of Spadina Avenue 🕓 Daily 🍴 Variety of eateries ($–$$) 🚇 St. Patrick 🚌 Dundas, Spadina or Bathurst streetcar

Ontario Place

Ontario Place is a popular summer amusement park located on the Toronto waterfront. Visitors can chose from 30 different rides, a huge water park called Soak City and Canada's largest soft-play climbing structure. There's the Rush River raft ride, a mega maze, bumper boats, the Mars Simulator ride and the wonderful Children's Village. A geodesic dome houses the Cinesphere, with an IMAX movie theater; the Molson Amphitheatre offers star-studded shows; and the Atlantis Pavilions have a nightclub that offers great views of Toronto's skyline from its rooftop patio.

www.ontarioplace.com

✚ *Toronto 1a (off map)* ✉ 955 Lakeshore Boulevard West ☎ 416/314-9900; 866/663-4386 (toll free) 🕓 Jun–Aug daily; May and Sep some weekends. Cinesphere, Molson Amphitheatre and Atlantis Pavilions: daily 🅿 Parking: very expensive 🍴 Restaurants ($–$$) 🚇 Union Station then streetcar 509 west to Exhibition; Bathurst, then streetcar 511 south to Exhibition Place; Wilson or Dufferin, then bus 29 south 🚆 GO Train to Exhibition Place 🚌 29; streetcars 509, 511 to Exhibition Place

Ontario Science Centre

A multimillion dollar project has made this world-leading science

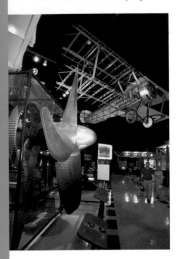

center even better, with an impressive range of 21st-century features that involve visitors of all ages. There are lots of fun "learn-through-play" areas for younger children, plus the inspirational Weston Family Innovation Centre that is designed to enthrall and challenge teens and young adults, from making music and fashion design to ecological problem-solving. There's also an OMNIMAX theater with a giant 24m (80ft) wraparound screen where you can be blown away by 13,000 watts of digital sound.

www.ontariosciencecentre.ca

✚ *Toronto 4f (off map)* ✉ 770 Don Mills Road ☎ 416/696-3127; OMNIMAX: 416/696-1000 ⏰ Daily 10–5 (to 6 in summer; extended hours for March Break); closed Dec 25 ✋ Expensive; parking charge: $8 🍴 Galileo's Bistro restaurant ($$–$$$), Lobby café and Valley Marketplace cafeteria ($) 🚇 Eglinton, then Eglinton bus 34 east or Pape, then Don Mills bus 25 ❓ Mastermind Toys gift store

Royal Ontario Museum

Already Canada's largest museum, the Royal Ontario Museum (ROM) now has a massive 7,500sq m (80,000sq ft) of additional exhibition space: The Michael Lee-Chin Crystal. Daniel Libeskind's stunning extension, inspired by the museum's mineral collection, is in the form of a giant crystal that bursts out of the original building in a riot of glass and metal prisms, angled over Bloor Street and up into the skyline.

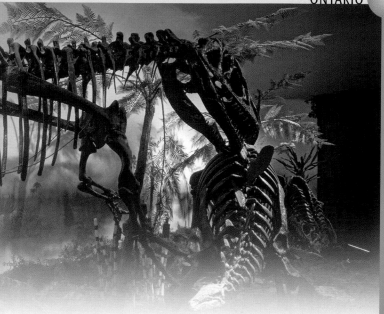

Inside, the breathtaking collections, amounting to some 6 million items, encompass world cultures from every continent and span the ages of civilization. Highlights include one of the foremost collections of Chinese temple art in the world, the excellent South Asia gallery and medieval European collections. Canada is also superbly represented, including a comprehensive insight into First Nations culture and the lives of the early European settlers.

The museum is also famous for its natural history collections, the most popular being the magnificent Age of Dinosaurs exhibit, which features 25 fully mounted skeletons and more than 300 other speciments, plus hundreds of fossils. Interactive information stations complete the fascinating insight into the past.

www.rom.on.ca

🕂 *Toronto 3f* ✉ 100 Queen's Park (main entrance on Bloor Street)
☎ 416/586-8000 🕓 Daily 10–5:30 (to 9:30pm Fri); closed Dec 25 and Jan 1
✋ Expensive; free after 4:30 Wed, half price Fri 4:30–9:30pm 🍴 Restaurant ($$$), cafeteria ($) 🚇 Museum ❓ Free guided tours daily. Gift store

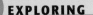

Toronto Islands

An urban oasis close to downtown Toronto, these islands provide a pleasant retreat from the summer heat of the city, as a light refreshing breeze blows in off the lake. For the visitor, they offer absolutely stunning views of the Toronto skyline, as well as beaches, picnic sites, walking and cycling trails, marinas, various sporting facilities and the Centreville amusement park and Franklin Children's Garden Farm for children.

Centre Island is the busiest area. From the ferry terminal here, it is about a 45-minute walk to either Hanlan's Point at the western end or to Ward's Island in the east. En route to Hanlan's Point, you will pass the Gibraltar Point Lighthouse which is reputedly the oldest surviving structure in Toronto (1806).

www.toronto.ca/parks/island

✚ *Toronto 4a (off map)* ☎ Toronto Parks: 416/392-1111 (general information); 416/397-2628 (island information line) 🕐 Daily (no winter ferry service to Centre Island) 🖐 Ferry fare: moderate 🍴 Rectory Café, Ward's Island ($–$$), seasonal snack bars ($), picnic sites 🚢 From foot of Bay Street to Hanlan's Point, Centre Island, and Ward's Island ☎ 416/392-8193 ❓ Bicycle rentals, public beaches

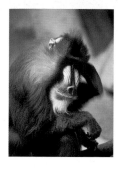

Toronto Zoo

Covering 287ha (710 acres), Canada's foremost zoo allows visitors to see animals from different areas of the world in settings that are as natural as possible. The African Savanna reserve is home to elephants, giraffes, antelopes and white rhinos, while a troop of gorillas provides entertainment in a separate pavilion. Kangaroos, wombats and pythons star in the Australasian enclosure, and in the Indomalayan pavilion is tropical forest with exotic birds and an orangutan family. The Canadian Domain houses native animals. There's also an interactive kids' zoo, Splash Island water park and entertainment at the Waterside Theatre.

www.torontozoo.com

✚ *Toronto 4f (off map)* ✉ Meadowvale Road, Scarborough ☎ 416/392-5929 🕐 Mid-Mar to mid-Oct daily 9–6 (to 7:30 mid-May to early Sep); mid-Oct to mid-Mar daily 9:30–4:30 ✋ Expensive. Parking charge Mar–Oct 🍴 Fast food ($), picnic sites 🚇 Kennedy then bus 86A; Don Mills then Sheppard East bus 85, 85A or 85B ❓ Zoomobile mini-train service around the zoo. Large animal-oriented gift store

Yorkville

Back in the 1960s, Yorkville was the center of the city's counter-culture. The rents were low and the drug culture prevailed. But times have changed, and it has now become Toronto's most

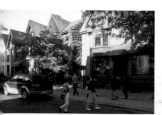

fashionable neighborhood with some of the most expensive real estate in Canada. Outdoor cafés flourish in the summer months and Yorkville and Cumberland avenues are packed with the rich and beautiful shopping in the *haute couture* boutiques and exclusive galleries.

✚ *Toronto 2f* 🚇 Bay

More to see in Ontario

ALGONQUIN PROVINCIAL PARK

Algonquin Provincial Park is the very essence of wilderness. Despite its location in central Ontario within a day's drive of both Ottawa and Toronto, the only way to explore the interior is by canoe or on foot. From the visitor center on Highway 60, a number of trails head for the interior. Algonquin offers splendid opportunities for viewing wildlife. White-tailed deer and bears can be seen, as can moose in spring, early summer and during the mating season. Algonquin is famous for its wolves, which are often heard but only rarely seen – in August, the park staff organize "wolf howling" expeditions. More than 260 species of bird have been recorded, including the common loon, which can be found nesting on just about every lake.

www.algonquinpark.on.ca

🚹 7C ✉ Box 219, Whitney, Ontario, K0J 2M0
☎ 705/633-5572 🕓 Daily 🍴 Food
services 👋 Inexpensive
❓ Accommodations
available, including
campsites

GEORGIAN BAY

Although it is part of Lake Huron, Georgian Bay is almost a lake in its own right thanks to the Bruce Peninsula and Manitoulin Island, which nearly enclose it. The southern part of the bay is blessed with sandy beaches where resorts proliferate. The northern and eastern shorelines are very indented; offshore here are thousands of small rocky islands of smooth granite topped with windswept trees. Scenic boat tours are available. The twin harbors at Tobermory, at the tip of the Bruce Peninsula, are full of pleasure craft in the summer months. A ferry crosses from here to Manitoulin Island. Just off Manitoulin is Flowerpot Island, famous for its picturesque sea stacks – visitors can take a cruise around the island and/or land and hike along its coast (4.3km/2.7 miles) to see these rock pillars.

www.georgianbaytourism.on.ca

➕ 6C ℹ️ 980 King Street, Midland, Ontario L4R 4K3 ☎ 800/263-7745
🚢 Ferry between Tobermory and Manitoulin Island (May to mid-Oct daily)
☎ 519/371-2354; 800/265-3163 (toll free) ✋ Access to Flowerpot Island: moderate. Boat cruises: expensive

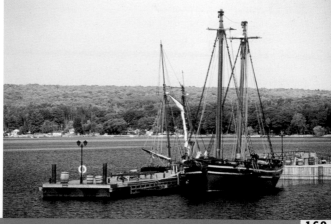

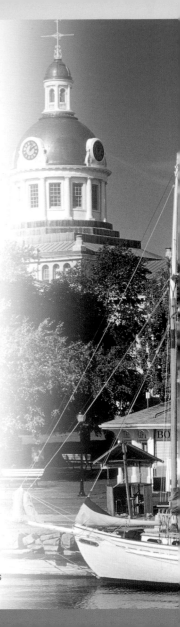

KINGSTON

Located at the eastern end of Lake Ontario, Kingston is a gracious city and is home to Queens University and the Royal Military College. Its grandiose City Hall was built in 1844 as a possible Parliament when the city hoped to become the capital.

An important British naval base in the early 19th century, it was equipped with a dockyard and an impressive stone fortress. Today restored to its full splendor, **Fort Henry** offers an excellent picture of military life in the mid-19th century, with barracks, kitchens, guard room and powder magazine, all animated by costumed interpreters and a trained troop who perform military displays.

www.kingstoncanada.com

✚ 8C 🛈 Kingston Tourist Information Office: 209 Ontario Street, Kingston, Ontario, K7L 2Z1 ☎ 613/548-4415; 888/855-4555 (toll free) ❓ Boats leave Kingston to cruise the Thousand Islands (➤ 176)

Fort Henry National Historic Site

www.forthenry.com

✉ County Road 2, P.O. Box 213, Kingston, Ontario, K7L 4V8 ☎ 613/542-7388 ☀ Mid-May to early Oct daily 10–5 👋 Expensive 🍴 Soldiers' canteen ($) ❓ Garrison Store (gift store); Fort Henry Guard sunset ceremonies: Wed, Jul–Aug (phone for details of other performances)

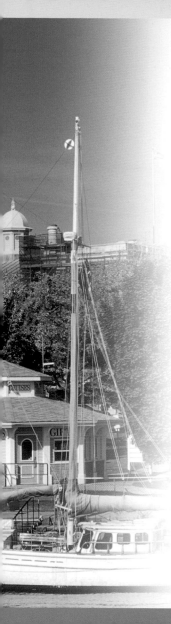

KLEINBURG

The small community of Kleinburg in the Humber River valley has the splendid **McMichael Canadian Art Collection** given to the province of Ontario by Robert and Signe McMichael. Located in a series of sprawling log buildings, the gallery is devoted entirely to Canadian art and features the finest collection in existence of works by the Group of Seven. In the 1920s, these artists sought to create a Canadian way of representing their country on its own terms rather than in the standard European tradition.

The galleries are arranged so that you can just ramble around admiring the works while at the same time looking out of the large windows at scenery similar to that depicted in the canvases. The McMichael also owns a superb collection of First Nations art, including sculptures by West Coast peoples, the striking prints of Norval Morrisseau and Inuit soapstone carvings.

www.kleinburgvillage.com

➕ 7B

McMichael Canadian Art Collection

✉ 10365 Islington Avenue, Kleinburg, Ontario L0J 1C0 ☎ 905/893-1121; 888/213-1121 (toll free); www.mcmichael.com ⏰ Daily 10–4; (to 5 Sun early May–late Oct); closed Dec 25 ✋ Expensive. Parking charge: $5 🍴 Restaurant ($$) ❓ Gallery shop

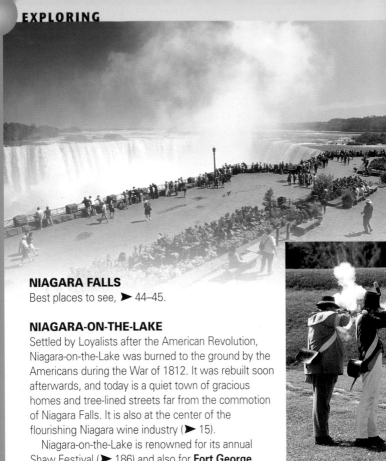

NIAGARA FALLS

Best places to see, ➤ 44–45.

NIAGARA-ON-THE-LAKE

Settled by Loyalists after the American Revolution, Niagara-on-the-Lake was burned to the ground by the Americans during the War of 1812. It was rebuilt soon afterwards, and today is a quiet town of gracious homes and tree-lined streets far from the commotion of Niagara Falls. It is also at the center of the flourishing Niagara wine industry (➤ 15).

Niagara-on-the-Lake is renowned for its annual Shaw Festival (➤ 186) and also for **Fort George.** Built in the 1790s, this garrison played an important role in the War of 1812 and has been restored to reflect that time.

www.niagaraonthelake.com

✚ 8B 🛈 Niagara-on-the-Lake Chamber of Commerce: 26 Queen Street, Niagara-on-the-Lake, Ontario, L0S 1J0 ☎ 905/468-1950

Fort George National Historic Park

✉ 26 Queen Street ☎ 905/468-4257; www.pc.gc.ca/lhn-nhs/on/fortgeorge
🕐 May–Oct daily 10–5, Apr and Nov Sat–Sun 10–5 🖱 Moderate
🍴 Restaurants in town ($–$$$)

NIAGARA PARKWAY

The Niagara Parkway follows the river on its course from Lake Erie to Lake Ontario. Put in place in 1923 by the Niagara Parks Commission, the parkway protects the environment around the falls from commercial development. Along its course drivers can enjoy the spectacle of the falls for themselves as well as more tranquil sections and the **Niagara Parks Botanical Gardens.**

At **Queenston Heights,** the Niagara Parkway crosses the Niagara Escarpment, a massive ridge of sedimentary rock towering 106m (350ft) above the river. The escarpment provides good soil and protection for the farmlands of the area.

www.niagaraparks.com

✚ 8B ✉ Niagara Parks Commission
🛈 Welcome Centers and information points at various locations ☎ 905/371-0254; 877/642-7275 (toll free)
Niagara Parks Botanical Gardens and Queenston Heights Park
☎ 905/371-0254 🕐 Daily 🖐 Free
🚌 Niagara People Mover bus (Mar–Dec)

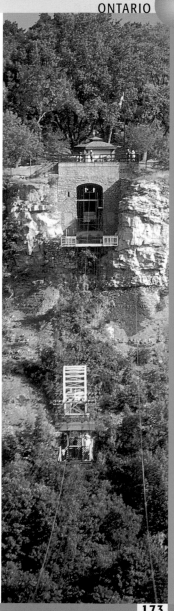

POINT PELEE NATIONAL PARK

At 42 degrees north (the same latitude as northern California and Rome), Point Pelee has a plant and animal life unique in Canada. This triangular peninsula in Lake Erie is what is known as a "migration trap." Thousands of birds and the monarch butterfly are among the creatures drawn here during the spring and fall migrations.

The Park Visitor Centre offers a wealth of information but be sure not to miss the special exhibit at Point Pelee (the most southerly tip of the Canadian mainland) that provides more information on bird migration.

www.pc.gc.ca/pn-np/on/pelee

✚ 6A ✉ 407 Monarch Lane, RR1, Leamington, Ontario, N8H 3V4 ☎ 519/322-2365; 888/773-8888 (toll free) ⊗ Daily 6am–10pm (7–7 Nov–Mar) ✋ Moderate 🍴 Cattail Café on the marsh boardwalk ❓ Tip of Canadian mainland accessible by private vehicle Nov–Mar; by free shuttle bus Apr–Oct. Bookstore in visitor center

SAULT STE. MARIE

"The Soo" is located on the north side of the St. Mary's River, which connects Lake Superior to Lake Huron. In just 1.5km (1 mile), this river drops more than 6m (21 ft) in a string of turbulent rapids (*sault* in French). Today, one of the busiest canal systems in the world is in place here, incorporating some of the world's longest locks (411m/1,350ft) so that shipping can make the passage. **Boat cruises** offer visitors the chance of viewing this last stage of the St. Lawrence Seaway, where ships complete their journey from the Atlantic into

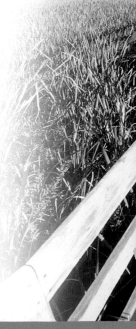

the heart of the continent. The Algoma railroad offers day trips into the wilderness to the north of Sault Ste. Marie (➤ 62).
www.saulttourism.com

✚ 5C ✉ Tourism Sault Ste. Marie: 99 Foster Drive, Sault Ste. Marie, Ontario, P6A 5X6 ☎ 705/759-5442; 800/461-6020 (toll free)

Lock Tours Canada Boat Cruises
✉ Roberta Bondar Park, Sault Ste. Marie ☎ 705/253-9850; 877/226-3665 (toll free); www.locktours.com 🕓 Late May–Sep daily 12:30 and 3 (also 6 late Jun–Aug); first 2 weeks in Oct daily 12:30 🖐 Expensive

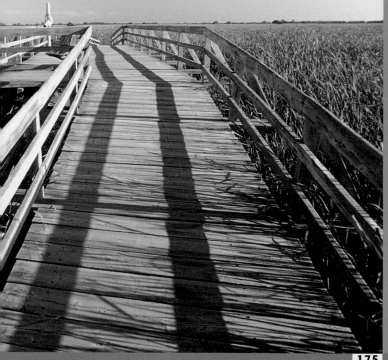

SUDBURY

Sudbury sits on the largest-known source of nickel and copper ores in the world. First and foremost a mining center, it is dominated by a 380m-high (1,250ft) chimney, known as "Super Stack." Most people make the trek to Sudbury to visit Science North (➤ 48–49), but there is also a fascinating mine to see here. **Dynamic Earth** is housed in the former Big Nickel Mine. An elevator transports you to the bottom of a rock chasm (20m/65ft down). As you descend, a presentation is projected onto the rock face. During the tour, former miners recount stories from Sudbury's mining history. At the surface, an exhibition center explains the importance of the crater in which Sudbury is located.

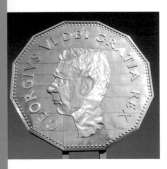

www.city.greatersudbury.on.ca
✚ 6C ✉ City of Greater Sudbury: Station A, 200 Brady Street, Sudbury, Ontario, P3A 5P3 ☎ 705/671-2489
Dynamic Earth
✉ 122 Big Nickel Road ☎ 705/523-4629; 800/461-4898 (toll free); www.dynamicearth.ca ⏱ Mid-Mar to late Apr daily 10–4; late Apr–late Jun daily 9–5; late Jun–early Sep daily 9–6 ✋ Expensive (combined ticket with Science North available)

THOUSAND ISLANDS

As it leaves Lake Ontario, the St. Lawrence River passes a multitude of islands, some large and forested, others simply rocky outcrops supporting a few pine trees. The exposed is Precambrian granite, with a pinkish hue in places, combined with the sparkling waters and surrounding greenery, makes this region delightful.
www.1000islandsgananoque.com
✚ 9C ✉ Chamber of Commerce, 10 King Street East, Gananoque, Ontario, K7G 1E6 ☎ 613/382-3250; 800/561-1595 (toll free)

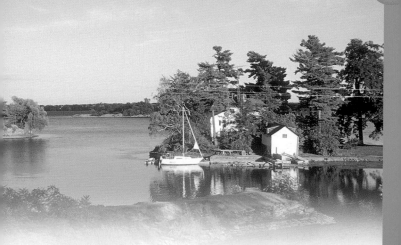

THUNDER BAY

Thunder Bay is located deep in the heart of the continent on the northwest shore of Lake Superior, at the head of navigation to the Great Lakes from the Atlantic. As such, it has been an important port and place of exchange. In the early 19th century, furs dominated the local economy, while most recently grain was handled here – huge elevators still dominate the skyline today.

The fur trade era is brilliantly recreated at **Old Fort William,** where you step back to the year 1815 when the canoes of the voyageurs filled the waterways, and a great rendezvous was held here every year to exchange pelts for trade goods. The reconstructed fort is huge, with more than 40 buildings, and is peopled by a whole cast of colorful characters.

www.visitthunderbay.com

✚ 3D

ℹ Tourism Thunder Bay, Terry Fox Centre, Highway 11–17, Thunder Bay, Ontario, P7C 5K4 ☎ 807/625-3960; 800/667-8386 (toll free)

Old Fort William Historical Park

✉ 1350 King Road, Thunder Bay, Ontario, P7K 1L7 ☎ 807/473-2344; www.fwhp.ca 🕓 Mid-May to mid-Oct daily 10–5 ✋ Expensive; moderate in May and Oct, when activities are reduced 🍴 Café ($) ❓ Trading Post gift store

UPPER CANADA VILLAGE

This imaginative and fun complex, located beside the St. Lawrence River, reproduces early life in what is now Ontario. It is not a museum as such, but a recreation of a slice of life as it was 150 years ago. At the time, this area of Ontario was settled by Loyalists, who worked hard to establish prosperous farms and businesses. While strolling round the village, you will meet the inhabitants as they go about their daily tasks such as cheese-making, tending livestock and spinning wool.

www.uppercanadavillage.com

🕇 9C ✉ 13740 County Road 2, Morrisburg, Ontario, K0C 1X0 ☎ 613/543-4328; 800/437-2233 (toll free) 🕐 Mid-May to early Oct daily 9:30–5 ✋ Expensive 🍴 Willard's Hotel ($$), Harvest Barn Restaurant ($), Village Café ($) ❓ Village Store – excellent Canadian gift shop

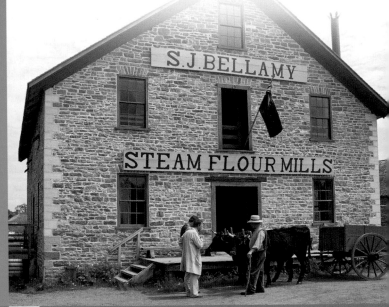

HOTELS

GANANOQUE
▼▼▼ Gananoque Inn ($$–$$$)
Historic inn with spectacular views beside the St. Lawrence. Rooms are located in several different buildings, some of them on the waterfront. Dining room with exceptionally good food.
✉ 550 Stone Street South ☎ 613/382-2165; 800/465-3101 (toll free); www.gananoqueinn.com

HAMILTON
▼▼▼ Visitors Inn ($$–$$$)
Above-average hotel in the city center. Rooms are stylish and some have kitchenettes. Indoor pool, fitness center; dining room.
✉ 649 Main Street West ☎ 905/529-6979; 800/387-4620 (toll free); www.visitorsinn.com

KINGSTON
▼▼ Peachtree Inn ($$)
Excellent location with easy access to the city, highways and shopping. Spacious rooms and loft-style suites.
✉ 1187 Princess Street ☎ 613/546-4411; 800/706-0698 (toll free); www.peachtreeinn.net

NIAGARA FALLS
▼▼▼▼ Sheraton Fallsview ($$$)
The best place in Niagara Falls – it is a high-rise structure with fabulous views of both the Canadian and American falls. Indoor pool, dining room (with views) and very high prices.
✉ 6755 Fallsview Boulevard ☎ 905/374-1077; 800/618-9059 (toll free); www.fallsview.com

NIAGARA-ON-THE-LAKE
▼▼▼▼ Pillar and Post Inn ($$$)
Lovely old inn (1890) in the heart of Niagara-on-the-Lake. Rooms are pleasantly Victorian in atmosphere. Full spa; excellent food.
✉ 48 John Street ☎ 905/468-2123; 888/669-5566 (toll free); www.vintage-hotels.com

OTTAWA
▽▼▽▼ ▽▼▽▼ Fairmont Château Laurier ($$$)

A magnificent château-style hotel in the heart of the capital. It is famous for the fact that the original table linen and silverware went down with the *Titanic*. Sports facilities and restaurant.

✉ 1 Rideau Street ☎ 613/241-1414; 800/257-7544 (toll free); www.fairmont.com/laurier

▽▼▽▼ Lord Elgin Hotel ($$$)

A city landmark just across the street from the National Arts Centre. For what it offers it is remarkably good value. Restaurant.

✉ 100 Elgin Street ☎ 613/235-3333; 800/267-4298 (toll free); www.lordelginhotel.ca

SAULT STE. MARIE
▽▼▽▼ Algoma Water Tower Inn ($$)

Motor inn on the north side of town with excellent facilities. Some rooms have wood-burning stoves and pine furniture. Good place for children, with sports facilities and Lone Star Restaurant.

✉ 360 Great Northern Road ☎ 705/949-8111; 800/461-0800 (toll free); www.watertowerinn.com

THUNDER BAY
▽▼▽▼ White Fox Inn ($$–$$$)

In a large wooded estate, just south of the city with views of the hills. Well-furnished rooms and the best food in the area.

✉ 1345 Mountain Road ☎ 807/577-3699; 800/603-3699 (toll free); www.whitefoxinn.com

TORONTO
▽▼▽▼ ▽▼▽▼ Fairmont Royal York ($$$)

A Toronto landmark, this huge hotel (nearly 1,400 rooms) is connected to the train station and the underground PATH system. Amazing lobby with chandeliers and handpainted ceiling. Elegant rooms and a indoor skylit pool and fitness center.

✉ 100 Front Street West ☎ 416/368-2511; 800/257-7544 (toll free central reservations); www.fairmont.com/royalyork 🚇 Union

▼▼▼ ▼▼▼ Windsor Arms ($$$)

South of busy Bloor Street, close to Yorkville and the University of Toronto campus. Luxury five-story hotel with tastefully furnished rooms. The Courtyard Café (▶ 182–183) is excellent.

✉ 18 St. Thomas Street ☎ 416/971-9666; 877/999-2767 (toll free); www.windsorarmshotel.com 🚇 Bay

RESTAURANTS

KINGSTON

▼▼▼ Chez Piggy ($$)

A downtown restaurant with a garden patio. Popular with the local literati from Queens University and the Royal Military College.

✉ 68R Princess Street ☎ 613/549-7673; www.chezpiggy.com 🕐 Daily 11:30am–midnight (from 11am Sun)

▼▼▼ The River Mill ($$–$$$)

The quintessential Canadian dining room, overlooking the Cataraqui River. Quiet, relaxed, and conservative.

✉ 2 Cataraqui Street ☎ 613/549-5759; www.rivermill.ca 🕐 Mon–Fri 11:30–2:30, from 5 for dinner, Sat dinner only. Closed Sun

NIAGARA FALLS

▼▼▼ Queenston Heights Restaurant ($$)

Relaxed, affordable restaurant overlooking the Niagara River; outdoor patio in summer. Far from the bustle of the falls.

✉ 14184 Niagara Parkway ☎ 905/262-4274; www.niagaraparks.com/dining/queenstonres.php 🍴 Early May–Jan lunch, dinner and Sun brunch. Hours vary. Closed Feb–early May

NIAGARA-ON-THE-LAKE

▼▼ Fan's Court ($$)

On the attractive main street. Very good Chinese cuisine inside or outside in a pretty courtyard in summer.

✉ 135 Queen Street ☎ 905/468-4511 🕐 Tue–Sun 12–9

OTTAWA
▽▽▽▽ Le Café ($$)
In the National Arts Centre overlooking the Rideau Canal. Pleasant outdoor terrace beside the canal in summer. Gourmet restaurant offering well-prepared Canadian specialties.

✉ 53 Elgin Street ☎ 613/594-5127; www.nac-cna.ca ⏰ Mon–Fri 12–11, Sat 5:30–11; winter: Mon–Fri 12–2, 5:30–11, Sat 5:30–11. Closed Sun

▽▽ Courtyard Restaurant ($$$)
Good Continental cuisine in an old stone building in a courtyard off Sussex Drive near the Byward Market (➤ 78).

✉ 21 George Street ☎ 613/241-1516; www.courtyardrestaurant.com ⏰ Mon–Sat 11:30–2, 5:30–9:30; Sun 11–2, 5–9

▽▽▽ Merlot ($$$)
Revolving restaurant atop the Marriott Hotel, with splendid views of the city and its site on the Ottawa River. Varied menu.

✉ 100 Kent Street ☎ 613/783-4212; www.merlotottawa.com ⏰ Mon–Sat 6pm–10pm, Sun 10:30–2, 6–10

SAULT STE. MARIE
▽▽▽ A Thymely Manner ($$)
In an old home. Uses only the best ingredients, herbs and spices for its menu of steak, pasta, and fish.

✉ 531 Albert Street East ☎ 705/759-3262; www.thymelymanner.com ⏰ Tue–Sat 5:30–11

TORONTO
▽▽▽ Bistro 990 ($$$)
French bistro that could be straight out of Paris. Serves excellent shrimp and filet mignon.

✉ 990 Bay Street ☎ 416/921-9990; www.bistro990.ca ⏰ Mon–Fri 12–10. Dinner only Sat and Sun 🚇 Wellesley

▽▽▽ ▽▽ Courtyard Café ($$$)
In the Windsor Arms Hotel near the University of Toronto campus. Luxurious restaurant with excellent rack of lamb and salmon, as

well as afternoon tea served in a relaxed atmosphere.

✉ 18 St. Thomas Street ☎ 416/971-9666; www.windorsarmshotel.com/cafe
🕐 Mon–Sat 7am–10 or 11pm, Sun brunch 10:30–2:30; closed Sun–Mon dinner 🚇 Bay

▼▼▼ ▼▼▼ Opus on Prince Arthur ($$$)

In a converted brownstone house close to Yorkville. Excellent Californian cuisine and an extensive wine list to choose from.

✉ 37 Prince Arthur Avenue ☎ 416/921-3105; www.opusrestaurant.com
🕐 Daily 5:30–11:30 🚇 St. George

▼▼ Pan on the Danforth ($$–$$$)

Upscale Greek dining with a rather eclectic menu. Good moussaka and a delicious casserole of chopped beef and potato.

✉ 516 Danforth Avenue ☎ 416/466-8158; www.panonthedanforth.com
🕐 Daily 12–11 (to midnight Fri–Sat) 🚇 Pape

▼▼▼ ▼▼▼ Scaramouche ($$$)

Just north of downtown. Romantic candlelit luxury, with splendid views of the Toronto skyline and acclaimed cuisine.

✉ 1 Benvenuto Place ☎ 416/961-8011; www.scaramoucherestaurant.com
🕐 Closed lunch and Sun 🚇 Summerhill

▼▼ Shopsy's Deli and Restaurant ($)

Shopsy's is a popular and noisy place close to the financial district with a huge menu of sandwiches, subs, soups and salads.

✉ 33 Yonge Street ☎ 416/365-3333; www.shopsys.ca 🕐 Mon–Wed 6:30am–11pm, Thu–Fri 6:30am–midnight, Sat 8am–midnight, Sun 8am–10pm
🚇 Union Station, King

SHOPPING

CENTERS AND MALLS
Canada One Factory Outlets

About 40 stores selling designer items with huge discounts, among them Liz Claiborne, Tommy Hilfiger and Ralph Lauren.

✉ 7500 Lundy's Lane, Niagara Falls ☎ 905/356-8989; 866/284-5781; www.canadaoneoutlets.com

Cataraqui Town Centre
Near the Trans-Canada Highway just west of the Cataraqui River. Has more than 140 stores, including The Bay, Zellers and Sears.

✉ 945 Gardiner Road, Kingston ☎ 613/389-7900; www.cataraquitowncentre.ca

Toronto Eaton Centre
See page 79.

MARKETS
Byward Market
See page 78.

Kensington Market, Toronto
See pages 162–163.

St. Lawrence Market
Historic market building housing more than 120 vendors, including artisan food producers, fruit and vegetables, bakeries, delicatessens, wine and crafts.

✉ 92 Front Street East, Toronto ☎ 416/392-7120; www.stlawrencemarket.com ⊗ Closed Sun–Mon ⊕ Union

CRAFTS AND OTHER SPECIALTIES
Algonquians Sweet Grass Gallery
Gallery owned by the Ojibwa. Exquisite sculptures in antler and soapstone, porcupine-quill jewelry and other traditional crafts.

✉ 668 Queen Street West, Toronto ☎ 416/703-1336 ⊕ Osgoode then streetcar 501 west ⊗ Usually closed Sun

Dr. Flea's
Covered market north of the city with about 400 vendors selling all manner of objects. Farmers' market in summer.

✉ 8 Westmore Drive, Toronto ☎ 416/745-3532; www.drfleas.com ⊗ Sat–Sun only ⊕ Royal York then bus 73

Fireworks
See glass artists and work and then buy their beautiful creations, from wine glasses and vases to ornaments and marbles.

✉ 56 Queen Street, Kingston ☎ 613/547-9149; www.glassrootsstudio.com

Eskimo Art Gallery
Large collection of Inuit soapstone sculpture on display in a gallery reminiscent of the Arctic, with iceberg and tundra decorations.

✉ 12 Queens Quay West, Toronto ☎ 416/366-3000; 800/800-2008 (toll free); www.eskimoart.com 🚇 Union then Harbourfront streetcar 509 or 510

Joyce Seppala Designs
Inspired by Canada's northern landscapes, Joyce Seppala designs stunning clothes in fleece fabrics that are both practical and fun.

✉ 508 East Victoria Avenue, Thunder Bay ☎ 807/624-0022; www.joyceseppaladesigns.com 🕐 Closed Sun

ENTERTAINMENT

CHILDREN'S ENTERTAINMENT
Lorraine Kimsa Theatre for Young People
Established in 1966, this excellent theater stages thought-provoking plays, musicals and comedy for children of various ages.

✉ 165 Front Street East, Toronto ☎ 416/363-5131; 416/862-2222 (box office); www.iktyp.ca 🚇 Union Station, King then streetcar east

Valleyview Little Animal Farm
Farm animals of all types, train ride and puppet shows (weather permitting). Best to visit in spring, when there are lots of baby animals to see. Café.

✉ 4750 Fallowfield Road, Nepean, Ottawa ☎ 613/591-1126; www.vvlittleanimalfarm.com 🕐 Mar–Oct Tue–Sun (also holiday Mons)

THEATERS AND NIGHTCLUBS
Elgin and Winter Garden Theatres
Beautifully restored theaters (the Elgin is downstairs, the Winter Garden above it) producing drama, music and comedy year-round.

✉ 189 Yonge Street, Toronto ☎ 416/314-2901 🚇 Queen

Four Seasons Centre for the Performing Arts

Toronto's magnificent modern opera house, which opened in 2006, was custom designed to host opera and ballet and is home to the Canadian national opera and ballet companies.

✉ 145 Queen Street West, Toronto ☎ 416/363-6671 (admin); 416/363-8231 (box office); www.coc.ca Ⓢ Osgoode

National Arts Centre

Performing arts center offering English and French theater, dance performances and classical and popular music shows year-round.

✉ 53 Elgin Street, Ottawa ✉ 613/947-7000; 866/850-2787 (toll free); www.nac-cna.ca

The Guvernment

Club complex on the waterfront offering big-name performers, local talent and DJs. Dress code for some shows.

✉ 132 Queens Quay East, Toronto ☎ 416/869-0045; www.theguvernment.com Ⓢ Union then walk east

Second City

The famous comedy club that has nurtured such internationally renowned talent as Mike Myers and Dan Ayckroyd.

✉ 51 Mercer Street ☎ 416/343-0011; 800/263-4485; www.secondcity.com Ⓢ Union Station

Shaw Festival Theatre

Theater primarily devoted to the production of the works of Irish writer George Bernard Shaw. The theater festival (Apr–Nov) also offers plays by other authors as well as comedy and musicals.

✉ 10 Queen's Parade, Niagara-on-the-Lake ☎ 905/468-2172; 800/511-7429 (toll free); www.shawfest.com

Stratford Festival of Canada

Canada's premier English-language theater company, producing the works of William Shakespeare and other classics (May–Nov).

✉ 55 Queen Street, Stratford ☎ 519/271-4040 (general enquiries); 800/567-1600 (box office); www.stratford-festival.on.ca

Sight Locator Index

This index relates to the maps on the covers. We have given map references to the main sights of interest in the book. Grid references in italics indicate sights featured on the town plans. Some sights within towns may not be plotted on the maps.

Index

Acknowledgements

The Automobile Association would like to thank the following photographers, companies and picture libraries for their assistance in the preparation of this book. Abbreviations for the picture credits are as follows: (t) top; (b) bottom; (c) centre; (l) left; (r) right; (AA) AA World Travel Library

4l Niagara Falls, AA/N Sumner; 4c Jeanne Marche Square, Montreal, AA/J F Pin; 4r Québec City, AA/N Sumner; 5l Biosphère, Montreal, AA/J F Pin; 5r Lake Memphremagog, AA/N Sumner; 6/7 Niagara Falls, AA/N Sumner; 8/9 Algonquin Provincial Park, AA/N Sumner; 10cl Parc du Mont Tremblant, AA/N Sumner; 10br Laurentides, AA/N Sumner; 10/11t Cape Breton Island, AA/N Sumner; 10/11c CBC Building Toronto, AA/J Davison; 11cr Virginia Deer, Laurentides, AA/J F Pin; 11c Montréal, AA/J F Pin; 11bl Whale, Nova Scotia, AA; 12/13t Lunenburg, AA/N Sumner; 12/13b PEI lobster supper, AA/N Sumner; 13tr Chocolates, AA/C Sawyer; 13cr Montréal, AA/J F Pin; 14 Seafood platter, AA/P Kenward; 15t Québec beer, AA/J F Pin; 15c Maple syrup sign, AA/C Coe; 15b Stratch Danial's Bar, Toronto, AA/J Beazley; 16 PEI lobster supper, AA/N Sumner; 16/17t Canadian beer, AA/J F Pin; 16/17b Chilliwack River, AA/P Timmermans; 18 Kensington Market, Toronto, AA/N Sumner; 18/19 Rogers Centre, AA/J F Pin; 19 Niagara Falls, AA/N Sumner; 20/21 Jeanne Marche Square, Montréal, AA/J F Pin; 22 Edwards Gardens, Toronto, AA/N Sumner; 24 Mounties, PEI, AA/N Sumner; 26 Lester Pearson International Airport, AA/J Beazley; 27 Montréal, AA/J F Pin; 28t Amtrak Adirondack, AA/R Elliot; 28c Canadian National Railways emblem, AA/J F Pin; 28b Old Montréal, AA/J F Pin; 29 Toronto taxi, AA/N Sumner; 34/35 Québec City, AA/N Sumner; 36 Museum of Civilization, AA/J F Pin; 36/37 Museum of Civilization AA/J F Pin; 37 Museum of Civilization, AA/J F Pin; 38/39 Gulf of St Lawrence, AA/J F Pin; 40/1 Toronto's waterfront skyline, AA/J F Pin; 41 CN Tower, Toronto, AA/N Sumner; 42/43 Montréal, AA/J F Pin; 44/45t Skylon Tower, Niagara Falls, AA/N Sumner; 44/45b Niagara Falls, AA/N Sumner; 46/47t Percé, AA/J F Pin; 46/47b Gaspé Peninsula boat trip, AA/J F Pin; 48/49 Science North Building, AA/N Sumner; 49 Science North Building, AA/N Sumner; 50 Cannon, St John's AA/N Sumner; 50/51 Cabot Tower, St John's, AA/N Sumner; 52 Musee de-la-Fort, Quebec, AA/N Sumner; 52/53 Terrasse Dufferin, AA/N Sumner; 53 Québec, AA/N Sumner; 54/55t Saguenay Fjord, AA/N Sumner; 54/55b Beluga Whales, Saguenay Fjord, AA/N Sumner; 56/57 Biosphère, AA/J F Pin; 59 Chateau Lake Louise, AA/P Bennett; 61 Halifax, AA/N Sumner; 62 Steam Train, Ottawa, AA/J F Pin; 65 Rogers Centre, AA/J Davison; 66/67 Ontario Place, AA/N Sumner; 68 Royal Ontario Museum Toronto, AA/J Davison; 69 Fisheries Museum of the Atlantic, Lunenburg, AA/N Sumner; 71 Lighthouse, Prince Edward Island, AA/N Sumner; 73 Bay Street, Toronto, AA/N Sumner; 74/72 Gros Morne National Park, AA/N Sumner; 76/77 Glasses and napkins, Stockbyte; 78 Eaton Center, AA/J Beazley; 80/81 Lake Memphremagog, AA/N Sumner; 83 Gros Morne National Park, AA/N Sumner; 84/85 Halifax, AA/N Sumner; 86l Citadel, Halifax, AA/N Sumner; 86r Sentry, Halifax, AA/N Sumner; 86/87 Halifax, AA/N Sumner; 88 HMCS Sackville, Halifax, AA/N Sumner; 89 Annapolis Royal, AA/N Sumner; 90/91 Bonavista Peninsula, AA/J F Pin; 93 Queen Street, Fredericton, AA/N Sumner; 92/93 City Hall, Fredericton, AA/N Sumner; 94 Fundy National Park, AA/N Sumner; 94/95 Gros Morne National Park, AA/N Sumner; 96/97 Innu Community of Davis Inlet, Bryan & Cherry Alexander Photography/Alamy; 98/99 Fortress Louisbourg, AA/N Sumner; 99 Fisheries Museum of the Atlantic, Lunenburg, AA/N Sumner; 100l Green Gables House, AA/N Sumner; 100r PEI National Park, AA/N Sumner; 101 St. Andrews, AA/N Sumner; 102 St. John's, AA/N Sumner; 102/103 Eagle, Terra Nova National Park, AA/N Sumner; 103 Terra Nova National Park, AA/J F Pin; 104 Acadian rug hooking, AA/J F Pin; 111 Horse and trap, Montréal, AA/J F Pin; 112 Montréal, AA/J F Pin; 112/113 Basilique Notre-Dame, AA/J F Pin; 114/115 Le Biodôme, AA/J F Pin; 115 Chapelle de Notre-Dame-de-Bonsecours, AA/J F Pin; 116/117 Jardin Botanique de Montreal, AA/J F Pin; 117 Musee d'Archeologie, AA/J F Pin; 118 Musee d'Art Contemporain, AA/J F Pin; 118/119 Habitat '67, Montréal, AA/J F Pin; 120 Montréal Underground, AA/J F Pin; 121 Parc Olympique, AA/J F Pin; 122/123 Place d'Armes, Montréal, AA/J F Pin; 123 Montréal, AA/J F Pin; 124/125t Québec City, AA/J F Pin; 124/125b Notre-Dame Basilica, AA/N Sumner; 126/127 Chateau Frontenac, AA/N Sumner; 128/129 Holy Trinity Anglican Cathedral, AA/N Sumner; 130t Place Royale, AA/J F Pin; 130b Promenade des Gouverneurs, AA/N Sumner; 131 Baie-Saint-Paul, AA/N Sumner; 132 Montmorency Falls, AA/J F Pin; 132/133 St-Benoit-du-Lac, AA/N Sumner; 134 St-Jean Manoir Mauvide-Genest, AA/N Sumner; 134/135 Île de Orleans, AA/J F Pin; 135 Bedroom, Saine-Jean Manoir Mauvide-Genest, AA/N Sumner; 136/137 Saint-Sauveur, AA/N Sumner; 137t Parc du Mont Tremblant, AA/J F Pin; 137b Ville Mont Tremblant, AA/N Sumner; 138 St-Rose-du-Nord, AA/N Sumner; 138/139 Ste-Anne-de-Beaupré Cathedral, AA/J F Pin; 139 Ste-Anne-de-Beaupré Basilica, AA/N Sumner; 140t Cap-de-la-Madeleine Shrine, Trois Rivieres, AA/N Sumner; 140b Musée des Ursulines, Trois Rivieres, AA/N Sumner; 149 Toronto, AA/J Beazley; 150 Rideau Canal, AA/N Sumner; 150/151 Ottawa, AA/N Sumner; 152/153 Canada Museum, Courtesy of Canada Aviation Museum 154 National Gallery, Ottawa, AA/J F Pin; 155 National Gallery of Canada, AA/N Sumner; 156 Parliament Hill, AA/N Sumner; 156/157 Rideau Canal, Ottawa Locks, AA/N Sumner; 158/159 Toronto at night, AA/N Sumner; 159t Toronto skyscrapers, AA/J Davison; 159b Art Gallery of Ontario, AA/N Sumner; 160 Fountain, Art Gallery of Ontario, AA/J Davison; 160/161 Flags, Art Gallery of Ontario, AA/N Sumner; 162/163 Kensington Market, AA/N Sumner; 164l Ontario Science Center, AA/J Davison; 164/165 Royal Ontario Museum, AA/J Beazley; 166 Hanlan's Point Beach, AA/N Sumner; 166/167 Hanlan's Point, AA/J Davison; 167t Metro Zoo, AA/N Sumner; 167b Yorkville, AA/J Davison; 168 Algonquin Provincial Park, AA/N Sumner; 169 Pentanguishene, AA/N Sumner; 170/171 Kingston, AA/N Sumner; 172 Niagara Falls, AA/N Sumner; 172/173 Fort Erie, AA/N Sumner; 173 Niagara Spanish Aero Cable Car, Niagara Parkway, AA/N Sumner; 174/175 Point Pelee National Park, AA/N Sumner; 176 Big Nickel, Sudbury, AA/N Sumner; 176/177 Thousand Island Parkway, AA/N Sumner; 178 Upper Canada Village, Stephen Saks Photography/Alamy.

Every effort has been made to trace the copyright holders, and we apologise in advance for any accidental errors. We would be happy to apply the corrections in the following edition of this publication.

Dear Reader

Your comments, opinions and recommendations are very important to us. Please help us to improve our travel guides by taking a few minutes to complete this simple questionnaire.

You do not need a stamp (unless posted outside the UK). If you do not want to cut this page from your guide, then photocopy it or write your answers on a plain sheet of paper.

Send to: **The Editor, AA World Travel Guides, FREEPOST SCE 4598, Basingstoke RG21 4GY.**

Your recommendations...

We always encourage readers' recommendations for restaurants, nightlife or shopping – if your recommendation is used in the next edition of the guide, we will send you a **FREE AA Guide** of your choice from this series. Please state below the establishment name, location and your reasons for recommending it.

_____

_____

_____

_____

_____

_____

Please send me **AA Guide** _____

About this guide...

Which title did you buy?

　　AA _____

Where did you buy it?_____

When? <u>m m</u> / <u>y y</u>

Why did you choose this guide? _____

_____

_____

_____

_____

Did this guide meet your expectations?

Exceeded ☐　Met all ☐　Met most ☐　Fell below ☐

Were there any aspects of this guide that you particularly liked? _____

_____

_____

_____

continued on next page...

Is there anything we could have done better? _____

_____

_____

_____

About you...

Name (*Mr/Mrs/Ms*) _____

Address _____

_____

_____ Postcode _____

Daytime tel nos _____

Email _____

Please only give us your mobile phone number or email if you wish to hear from us about
other products and services from the AA and partners by text or mms, or email.

Which age group are you in?
Under 25 ☐   25–34 ☐   35–44 ☐   45–54 ☐   55–64 ☐   65+ ☐

How many trips do you make a year?
Less than one ☐   One ☐   Two ☐   Three or more ☐

Are you an AA member? Yes ☐   No ☐

About your trip...

When did you book? m m / y y   When did you travel? m m / y y

How long did you stay? _____

Was it for business or leisure? _____

Did you buy any other travel guides for your trip? _____

If yes, which ones? _____

_____

_____

Thank you for taking the time to complete this questionnaire. Please send it to us as soon as
possible, and remember, you do not need a stamp (*unless posted outside the UK*).

┌───┐
│ **AA** Travel Insurance call **0800 072 4168** or visit **www.theAA.com** │
└───┘